MW01096764

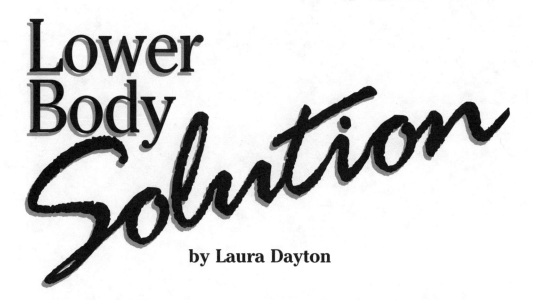

Lower Body Solution

by Laura Dayton

Pare down the "pear" shape with this new exercise plan to lose the stubborn fat that other programs can't touch

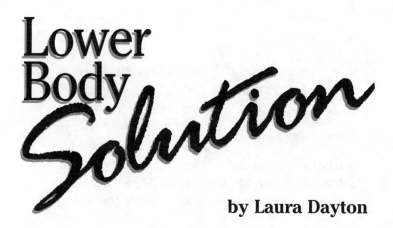

Lower Body Solution

by Laura Dayton

A one-day-at-a-time program to shed the stubborn fat that plagues women and seems utterly resistant to exercise and diet. Diet tips. Supplements that burn fat. And an awesome exercise program for women-only that works on every size, age and shape.

Editor:	Kim David Goss, C.S.C.S.
Assistant Editor:	Deborah Ryan
Art Director:	Caron Gordon
Exercise Photography:	Laura Vitale
Copy Editor:	Christine Bettencourt
Administrative Assistant:	Suzy Solomon
Exercise model:	Veronica Chojnacki

DAYTON PUBLICATIONS
1541 Third St., Napa, CA 94559
(707) 257-2348   fax: (707) 257-2349
e-mail: Daytonpubs@aol.com

*A*s a former Mr. America, and having spent ten years billed as "the world's greatest strongman," I have made weight training my passion, my career and in many ways my life. Yet I take a back seat to a woman who knows far more about weight training than I: my sister Laura Dayton.

It's not the first time she's changed the way women exercise; however, it may be the last: this program is so incredibly thorough and easy to follow, it may put personal trainers out of business!

Mike Dayton
1976 Mr. America

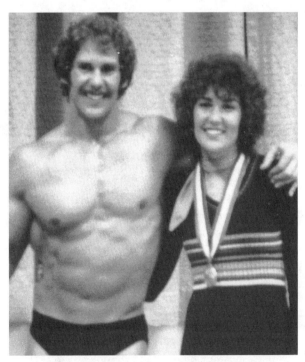

Mike Dayton and sister Laura in 1976 on the night he won the professional Mr. America title.

Table of Contents

What's Wrong?
Why Nothing Seems to Work

We sweat and fret about our weight. Over the past 25 years there have been hundreds of magazines and thousands of articles about fitness and weight loss. I know. I wrote many of them.

Despite this information overload we as a nation, and women in particular, are getting fatter than ever. Sure, some women manage to look fabulous even after childbirth and/or hitting age 40. But a quick visit to the beach or poolside offers tons of bulging, drooping evidence of just how poorly most programs work for most women.

The problem is threefold:
- **First**, women have only been seriously exercising for a few decades, and it's taken this long for effective techniques to evolve.
- **Secondly**, exercise has been approached from a unisex standpoint that doesn't adequately address a woman's needs. Women gain and lose fat differently than men and need a unique approach.
- **Lastly**, female fat has become more stubborn than ever!

This book is the culmination of nearly 30 years spent writing, researching and discussing weight loss. To my knowledge, it is the most complete and universal approach ever offered to women. It's flexible enough to fit anyone's lifestyle, even the busiest of moms and/or career women. It has worked on a variety of women from age 17 to 76, having anywhere from 5 to 170 pounds to lose. It's worked for me, and now it's going to work for you.

Are You Exercising Wrong?

It's a fact that Americans are fatter than ever, despite a nearly zealous no-fat diet craze in the past ten years. It's also a fact that women devote a tremendous amount of time, effort and mental anguish trying to improve their physical appearance. Still, for most of us, that ideal body seems to be hopelessly out of reach.

Surrounded by stick-thin models and actresses, not to mention photos of 50-something Raquel Welch still looking like a 20-something *Baywatch* babe, women are understandably dissatisfied with their bodies. This book isn't about turning you into a 98-pound twig; it is about getting your weight down and under control. It's about becoming stronger and healthier, and feeling better about yourself. It will explain why most programs fail. It will present you with a unique and precise program that has been proven to change the shape you're in and take off weight. It's about an exercise routine that really and truly works for women.

Following the *Lower Body Solution* program will

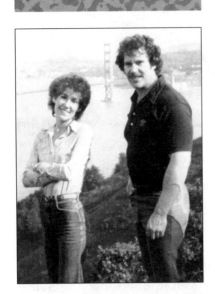

This was taken in 1978 when my brother's career as a strongman was just beginning. Weighing a mere 98 pounds at the time, I was already quite prolific as a ghostwriter for my brother and several other prominent body-builders of the era. Little did anyone know the person telling guys how to build 22-inch arms had 12-inch biceps!

lower your overall body fat, especially in the hips, thighs and low belly. However, fat will melt from all parts of your body: your back, cheeks, chin and arms as well. Physiologically, women are pro-grammed to store an abundance of fat in regions of the lower body, making these areas especially difficult to slim. This book will show you an innovative way to shave extra inches off your nether regions, even if you're from a family of disproportionately large lower bodies. One woman even had to quit the program because she felt her thighs and rear were getting too small!

Part of the reason exercise programs haven't worked for you in the past is that you were doing the wrong exercise program. How do I know this? Well, the fact that you're reading this book is my first hint. Also, the fact that everything women have been taught to do, as it pertains to exercise, has been from a man's perspective.

I remember when there was literally no such thing as a coed gym and, at 46, I'm not *that* old. Men had gyms with weights and equip-ment; women had studios or salons with mats on the floors, a sta-tionary bike or two and maybe one of those machines with wooden rollers that was suppose to "heat" your fat and "melt" it off. If you look in dictionaries from the 1970s you'll notice the word "aerobics" wasn't even included!

The late seventies ushered in a new enthusiasm for aggressive exercise, and women en masse began exercising seriously. Most importantly, women began lifting weights. The programs they fol-lowed were the same routines as men but with lighter weights and, sometimes, longer aerobic sessions. Trainers agreed that a muscle was a muscle, and while women may lift lighter weights, everyone agreed that women and men should follow the same program.

That was wrong. I don't mean to insult those personal trainers and exercise experts, but their approach to exercise for women has been all wrong. I don't want to insult them because I was one of them. It took me many years of doing things wrong to begin to figure out how to do them right.

Been There, Done That

My earliest encounters with exercise came in the 1950s when "Uncle" Jack LaLanne appeared on the old black and white Motorola and told all us "kiddies" to "run and get your moms." I did, and even managed a few fire hydrant kicks and sit-ups with mom back in those days.

As I matured into an adolescent in the 1960s, I had my nose buried in the pages of *Young Mr. America* magazine while other girls my age were playing with Barbie. Long before the days of Arnold I could name every top physical culturist (as they called bodybuilders back then) along with those circus strongmen who bent bars in their teeth. I admit that may sound a little weird.

The weird guy was actually my brother Mike, four years older than I, who aspired to be a circus strongman. He would do push-ups with me and my youngest brother lying on his back. Mike loved anything that was odd and out of the ordinary. I remember watching as my then-60-pound little brother would stand on Mike's open palm and be lifted overhead at arm's length (with considerable strength on Mike's part) where he would preen triumphantly, arms outstretched like a gymnast after a perfect dismount. Of course, we had to do this particular feat outside where there was no ceiling impediment, and also a soft surface for the failed attempts. Whether he made the lift or dropped my brother face-first in the dirt, I was always there to cheer on the performance.

The three of us turned our basement rumpus room into a mini circus, and staged performances where Mike would perform 50 push-ups, rip apart phone books and pose like the bodybuilders in the magazines. At age 18 Mike actually became the youngest ever to win the Teenage Mr. America title. I was the proudest little sister in the world, and already his biggest fan.

Growing up with three brothers (there was a fourth who never followed us into the bodybuilding scene) made it easy for me to live in the world of bigger-than-life Marvel Comics superheroes instead of Archie and Veronica. The only doll I ever owned was beheaded during a raucous game of Zorro by my brothers and me in the backyard. Eventually, however, we all grew up. As I hit my teenage years I found new friends, shaved my legs, discovered makeup, then boys. Needless to say, I quit reading bodybuilding magazines.

Oh, did I say we all grew up? Whoops. I should say, more correctly, most of us grew up.

Fueled by his win of the Teenage Mr. America title, my brother went on not only to become Mr. America, but also to perform a strongman act that won him spots on the *Merv Griffin Show, That's Incredible* and several other television shows. He never actually worked in a circus, but he snapped baseball bats in two and broke out of police handcuffs to the cheers of packed houses at bodybuilding shows and on European tours. He is still featured on ESPN in segments from a 1977 World's Strongest Man Contest.

While my brother was carving his rather unique career niche, I was finishing up my college degree in journalism. I had lost count of the rejection letters I received while trying to get my first article published when I realized that bodybuilding magazines were clamoring for articles and information on my brother, who now was being called the World's Greatest Strongman. I had an "in" and started ghostwriting articles for Mike.

During my high school and early college years I was as skinny as a toothpick. Aside from softball in the backyard—there were no team sports in school for girls then—my only sporting activity was bowl-

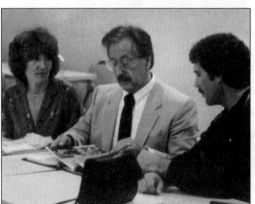

I first met Joe Weider, publisher of Muscle and Fitness *in 1981. Joe would later introduce his highly successful* Shape *magazine at a time when I was working on its rival,* Fit *magazine. Here my brother and I shared our own publication,* Natural Bodybuilding, *with the most powerful man in the sport of bodybuilding.*

ing. As I began to write articles under my brother's name, my interest in exercise grew, and when the first coed health clubs began to spring up I was one of the first to sign up.

My interest in exercise, and my article writing, both increased at a fast pace. My first article was published in 1971 in *Ironman* magazine, and it was quickly followed by a series. I wrote columns, features and training articles under a variety of names, some fictitious, some by other bodybuilders. I managed to supplement my income in this way as I put myself through graduate school.

In 1979 my brother and I began publishing a magazine called *Natural Bodybuilding*. This innovative magazine was the first to rally against athletic steroid use, and also the first to cover a new sport: women's bodybuilding.

In 1984 when the publisher of *Runner's World* magazine wanted a woman editor for a new magazine about this budding sport, I got the job. The magazine was called *Strength Training for Beauty*, and it helped shape the sport of female bodybuilding. Its covers featured Rachel McLish, Cory Everson, Marjo Selin and countless others who would gain fame as the sport springboarded in popularity. It eventually spawned a full-length feature film, *Pumping Iron II*, and coverage on CBS.

All things must pass, as did the sport of women's bodybuilding, and rather quickly I might add. However, personally, that launching pad led to more freelance and editorial positions for me at dozens of other fitness and bodybuilding magazines, including the editorships of *Fit* and *Women's Fitness* magazines. Sometimes I wrote under my name, sometimes under someone else's. If you have read a fitness or bodybuilding magazine over the past 28 years, you have most likely read my routines, training and diet advice.

I'm sharing this with you so that you realize I'm not clairvoyant when I say that you've been exercising wrong. I can say that because I'm one of the people who were giving you bad advice. When I look back at my early writing and some of the things I used to believe were exercise doctrine, I shudder.

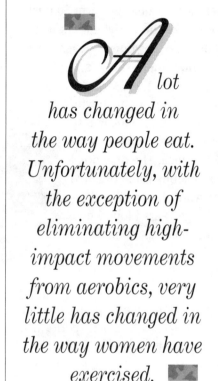

A lot has changed in the way people eat. Unfortunately, with the exception of eliminating high-impact movements from aerobics, very little has changed in the way women have exercised.

Sorry, I didn't know any better. And it seems neither did quite a few other "experts."

Over these years I have amassed quite a collection of health and fitness books that I use for reference. I find it amazing that in Adelle Davis' 1970 bestseller *Let's Eat Right to Keep Fit*, there is no mention of fiber among necessary nutrients. As a matter of fact, it is not even a nutrient. Do you think the government was any better? The 1968 Recommended Daily Allowances (RDA) list for vitamins and nutrients underwent 55 changes in values from the 1964 list, with variations from 20 to 700 percent. A similar revision was made in 1974. No wonder some people claim RDA stands for "ridiculous, dangerous and arbitrary." Remember in 1990 when they turned the food chart upside down? After being raised on a "meat, milk and eggs" mentality we suddenly learn that whole grains, fruits and vegetables should compose the majority of our diet, with significant limitations on meat and dairy.

A lot has changed in the way people eat. Unfortunately, with the exception of eliminating high-impact movements from aerobics, very little has changed in the way women have exercised over the past 20 years.

For women, this book will change all that.

Bodybuilding vs. Weight Training

I know that most women today do not want to look like a bodybuilder. It's repulsive. This book isn't about bodybuilding, but it is about weight training. Understanding a little about the evolution of the sport will help you make the very important distinction between bodybuilding and weight training.

The sport of women's bodybuilding wasn't always gross. At first, it was fun and the results attractive. It was more than a sport; it was a movement. Right in the midst of the Gloria Steinem days when women were calling for equal rights and equal pay, and demanding a place alongside men in the workplace and in government, here we were boldly walking through the doors of once totally male bastions. Not only were we taking over male gyms, we were training right alongside the guys on the weights. We were the "Ladies of the Eighties" and the sport of women's bodybuilding soon emerged.

What a blast those early days were! Most of us were barely out of our rebellious teenage years and leading a revolution of strong, sexy women. Biceps got bigger and body fat was slashed. We were strong and confident. Why put shoulder pads in silk blouses when we could build our own? The new curves were sexy and attractive, and enviable as everyone from Jane Fonda to Madonna began working out with weights in earnest.

Weight training also produced immediate results. Strength was gained with every workout. Our bodies changed. It was wonderful to take control of a body that through most of puberty was loaded with surprises. Now, we were masters of our physical beauty. If you weren't born with a body endowed with perfect Miss America genetics, you could go to a gym and change it. We were empowered and it was a magical time.

Many times in my magazines I would ask the rhetorical questions: "How far can it go? How strong can we become? How big can we grow?"

Unfortunately, the answers to those questions came all too soon, and bodybuilding's "Ladies of the Eighties" never made it to the nineties.

It should have come as no surprise that when women were put in the same kind of competitive environment as men—an environment that required them to build the largest muscle possible—that women would also resort to any and every means to accomplish that goal. Following the lead of male bodybuilders, women began taking steroids and other growth agents, and they began quite literally to turn into men. Little was known about long-term steroid use and next to nothing was known about women taking steroids. At first the changes were exciting, but it wasn't long before it turned into a freak show.

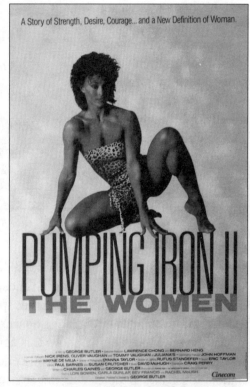

A Story of Strength, Desire, Courage... and a New Definition of Woman.

PUMPING IRON II
THE WOMEN

Women's bodybuilding reached its zenith with the release of Pumping Iron II: The Women. *The movie portrayed a battle between the bodybuilders who were "big and beefy" and those who were "sleek and sexy." Mirroring life, the movie, as did the general public, picked sleek and sexy as the more desirable look for women.*

Most women are not born with enough testosterone naturally occurring in their bodies to build the 170-pound-plus, 7-percent body fat physiques of professional women bodybuilders in the 1990s. Women can certainly build muscle naturally, but the really huge displays of muscle on professional female bodybuilders are a product of steroid use.

What was known back in the 1980s was that if a man is injected with estrogen he will temporarily exhibit female traits, such as breasts. Once the hormones are discontinued, his body will go back to its masculine state. What was not known back then was that if a woman is given male hormones such as steroids, she will become permanently masculinized. Sure, some of the effects will diminish when steroid use is discontinued, but not all. I know many women who still have full, dark beards from steroid use. I know one woman who told me her clitoris grew to a record length of four inches using steroids. I know countless women who now possess a baritone voice. Those were the kinds of stories that drove the sport of women's bodybuilding into relative obscurity.

(Like Jerry Springer's TV show, this aspect of women's bodybuilding holds a certain odd fascination for many people. For this reason I've reprinted one of my articles on the subject in the back of this book. Its publication several years ago created the biggest stir of any of my articles, even a phone call from *Hard Copy*, so I felt this would be an appropriate place to reprint it for reference on the subject of women and steroid use.)

The worst tragedy to come out of the sport of women's bodybuilding was that some women permanently altered their secondary sexual characteristics in pursuit of a plastic trophy. However,

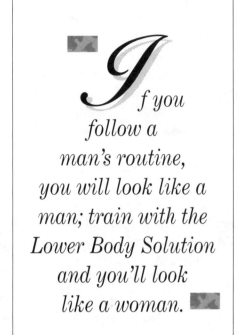

If you follow a man's routine, you will look like a man; train with the Lower Body Solution and you'll look like a woman.

just as tragic is the fact that when women began using steroids, the rest of the world wrinkled their noses in disgust at the entire idea of women and weight training. This is such a shame, because there is nothing wrong with muscle tone, strength and athletic ability in a woman. A female bodybuilder baring her teeth and clenching her fists in a "crab pose" is something entirely different, even though both are a result of weight training.

This distinction—that weight training does not have to result in the large muscular displays of bodybuilders—has been hard for many people to make. With the sheer freakishness of some of today's professional bodybuilders, I don't blame women for being utterly afraid of weights. But the fear is unfounded.

Nonetheless, in the 1990s women turned away from weight rooms and hightailed it back to the safe sanctuary of the aerobics studio. If they did weight train, it was only a minor part of their routines. Instead, women have been enjoying cardio-funk, hip-hop, boxercise, spinning and dozens of other aerobic exercise programs. This is part of the reason we are getting fatter! Aerobics may work for a time, but when they are the sole source of exercise they too often fail to keep a woman's weight under control!

We now know that most women do not want big muscles. We also know that weight training can cause big muscles. What most people don't know is that there are ways to weight train that do not create large muscles. Further, there is a way to use weight training to lose weight that is more effective than aerobics alone. It is the only way to effectively gain control of a body that is genetically predisposed to weight gain and a midlife figure going through the chemical changes of menopause. Weight training in this fashion is what the *Lower Body Solution* is about.

Manly Exercise: What You <u>Don't</u> Want to Do

Weight training began as a way for male athletes to become stronger. It evolved into a sport: bodybuilding. The bodybuilding mentality, like a flesh-eating disease, completely consumed the fitness and health club industry. Those involved in the sport of bodybuilding perfected a way to build the body through weight training. It involves certain principles:

1. The total body is defined as five main body parts: arms/shoulders, back, chest, abs, legs.
2. Each of these body parts requires equal attention for a balanced physique.
3. Two to three exercises for three sets of ten repetitions per body part is the norm.
4. Always allow at least two days' rest for each body part for recuperation, which is necessary for growth.

These criteria, when diligently followed, will build manly-looking muscle. When you walk into almost any health club in the world you will be given a program that meets these general criteria, even if manly muscle is not your goal. When you read the instructions preprinted on machines, in magazines and posted on health club walls, you will read these principles as though they were gospel.

What I'd like to know is who says these principles are right?

A friend of mine once researched the literature in order to find the scientific study that advised drinking eight glasses of water a day as the ideal amount of water we should consume. She came up empty-handed, except for an obscure study of 28 European athletes who performed better on eight glasses of water. Yet, eight glasses of water has become a magical number representing an adequate amount of water we should all consume. In the same way, we have all assumed that following a basic bodybuilding approach to weight training is the proper way to weight train. True for the bodybuilder, but not for the average woman.

While extensive studies have been conducted in the U.S. on aerobic exercise, relatively little exists on exercise as it affects women. The Europeans are far more advanced than we are in that regard. However, even in European journals the "a muscle is still a muscle" attitude prevails regardless of whether it's on a man or a woman.

It's true that all muscles react to exercise the same. Where everyone seems to have missed the boat is that men and women desire

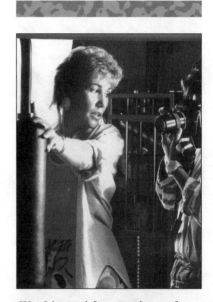

Working with a variety of magazines and photographers in the 1980s gave me the chance to work with, and become friends with, many of the bodybuilding and the fitness field's biggest celebrities. Many of these people, including Rachel McLish, Cory Everson and Karen Voight, have helped shape my opinions about exercise and training.

drastically different results from that exercise. Consider these:

- **Men want a big, thick, hard chest.**
- *Women want attractive and firm breasts.*
- **Men want big arms.**
- *Women want an attractive shoulder curve and triceps that don't flap in the wind.*
- **Men want muscle, strength and size.**
- *Women want tone and low body fat.*
- **Men want a rock-hard body like Sylvester Stallone's.**
- *Women want a cellulite-free figure like Sharon Stone's.*

This discovery, simple as it seems now, was one that came about only after I was able to step away from the bodybuilding and gym-rat mentality and look at fitness as an "outsider."

As I've told you, for most of my adult life my circle of friends have been fitness fanatics. My stick-thin genetics always kept me from getting huge muscles (although at one time I could bench press 135 pounds), yet I always stayed in better-than-average shape. I thought nothing of going to the gym six days a week. I did notice the club was empty on Friday nights, but it hadn't occurred to me that I didn't have a life.

At the unlikely age of 41, and against the odds according to *Cosmopolitan* magazine, I fell head-over-heels in love. That part was strange enough, but my big and buffed friends found it even stranger that my husband-to-be had never read a bodybuilding magazine in his life. We had other things in common like skating, skiing and sailing. While he had a definite interest in staying lean and healthy, fitness wasn't the only thing in his life. Far from it! At the time I met him he was playing Mr. Mom full-time to his two kids.

A year later I was, for the first time in my life, driving kids to school, attending soccer games, shopping at discount bulk food stores and skipping my workouts in order to cook dinner for people who didn't think a grilled skinless chicken breast and raw broccoli constituted a meal. I might add, I was having the time of my life. I still went to work where I wrote and spoke about fitness for eight hours a day, but my new world exposed me to a gamut of people who didn't swig protein shakes with carrot juice chasers and didn't live for keeping their bodies hard, firm and free of fat. I had finally come in intimate social contact with the very people I had spent a good deal of my career writing for: average, middle-America women.

I confess to once believing that overweight and frustrated women were the way they were because they didn't care. As I came to know them I realized they did care; they simply didn't know how to change. I also saw that most of the information coming from the fitness industry, including that coming from me, was of little use to them.

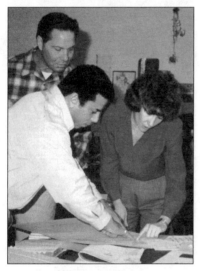

In addition to working with the sport's female elite, I have also rubbed elbows with many of the top male bodybuilders. Here I'm discussing a layout with former Mr. Olympia Chris Dickerson and bodybuilding's most amiable and respected superstar, Mr. Bill Pearl.

The fitness industry, with its attitude that spending your life in the gym is a perfectly normal, even superior, way to live, let these women down. I began to see excess weight gain not as something caused by a character deficiency, but as a natural process that befalls most American women. I began to make some radical changes in the way I pitched and preached fitness.

Weight Training for Weight Loss

About this time I co-authored an article with a man who had worked for me back at *Runner's World*, Kim Goss. In the time since he'd left *Runner's World*, Kim had put in eight successful years as a strength coach at the Air Force Academy in Colorado Springs, coaching 27 different varsity sports. Also under his tutelage were some top-ranked figure skaters—young girls who faced the dilemma of having to build and maintain strength through weight training but stay physically slim and unmuscular. From that experience Kim and I wrote an article entitled "The German Body Shaping Program," which was published in *Cross Trainer* magazine in 1994 and was the first program to promote weight training for weight loss without a gain in muscle size. It was the most popular article ever published in the magazine, demonstrating that not all men want to build large muscle either.

For nearly a year Kim and I worked on the concepts of weight training for weight loss, aided by invaluable contributions from Canadian strength coach extraordinaire, Charles Poliquin. Nearly 20 years after my first article was published I wrote my first book, *Freestyle Training*, which promoted a radically different approach to women's weight training than I had preached in *Strength Training for Beauty*. Instead of promoting bodybuilding, *Freestyle Training* offered a method whereby women could weight train without gaining size.

Kim was now working with me full-time, and while the fitness writing business had been good for more than two decades, after *Freestyle* was published things really began to take off. We began ghostwriting for some of the biggest names in sports and the fitness industry, while sharing their vast knowledge and experience in the process. We were producing the majority of information in three newsstand publications and began publishing all of Coach Poliquin's books. Charles has coached literally thousands of athletes to gold, silver, bronze, world, national and personal best records. His exhaustive research in the field of strength training has set new precedents for athletic protocols. His knowledge and input were integral in developing the *Lower Body Solution* program.

My book *Freestyle Training* presented the tip of the iceberg with its women-only approach to weight training. But three years later, at age 45, I realized the program couldn't work forever and was limited to very young women and those with only a few pounds to lose. I had

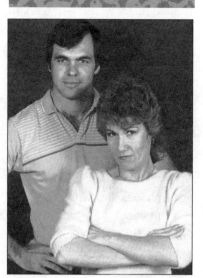

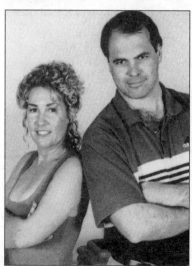

Fifteen years apart and you can hardly see a difference? Yeah, right! The top photo of coach Kim Goss and me was taken for an editorial in 1983. The second photo was taken just a few months ago.

personally made many modifications over the years to my own *Freestyle*-based training. I'd also trained many women—mostly my age and older—on the program, always modifying as I went. I had learned a lot, and knew there was still more to learn. And who better to practice on than myself, someone who had grown into a slightly overweight, middle-aged wife and stepmom who had found better things to do than spend 20 hours a week in the gym!? If I could devise a program that would work for me, I knew it would work for other busy moms (and stepmoms) and women of all ages, shapes and sizes.

I threw out a few of the original premises of my *Freestyle Training* book and started anew. I tapped my resources of 28 years in the fitness industry to help me devise a workout and a diet plan that would make a radical reduction in the amount of fat a woman carries—not just on her lower body, although that was my primary emphasis, but overall.

I realized that I needed to write another book. It needed to be a book for real women in their 30s, 40s, 50s, 60s and even older. A book for women 5, 50, 100 or more pounds overweight. A book with a program based on sound, state-of-the-art science. A book for women who have a life (mate, kids, family) and that doesn't assume you want to (or can) devote all your free time to the gym. A book with a program that truly fights age-induced weight gain. A book with a program that offers a real solution to a woman's lower body weight gain. A book that reflects all I have learned in this field, and especially since the publication of *Freestyle Training*. A book that shares my own struggle with middle-age weight gain, and my successful strategy to beat it.

This is that book.

Success Stories

Something is about to happen. At the very least you are going to give some honest thought to the shape you're in. At the very best you will embrace lifestyle changes that will beautify your body and add years of energetic living to your life.

Exactly how this program will enrich your life is a chapter only you can write. However, I can share with you many true stories of how this same program has created changes both large and small in other women's lives. In these stories you may find parallels that will help you form realistic expectations and goals.

Emotional Fitness

I know you want to flip forward and dive right into the *Lower Body Solution*. Before you do, I hope you take the time to read this very important chapter. It's important because the stories tell the emotional side of weight loss and getting in shape. I believe that for most men, getting in shape is merely an exercise drill: read the routine, lift the weights. Women are different creatures. We are emotional, and I for one can relate to new ideas far better when I understand the feelings involved. The stories in this chapter explore many of the emotions that are tied into getting in shape.

I also believe that approaching a shape-up pro-

gram purely from the "sets and reps" perspective is why many women fail. Our society's preoccupation with how women look has distorted our self-images. There is hardly a woman alive who is happy with the shape she is in, no matter how perfect she looks! Being out of shape is a source of incredible frustration, embarrassment and sadness. Getting in shape can also be a source of incredible frustration, embarrassment and sadness. We need to acknowledge that these feelings may be part of the process. Too many people approach fitness without considering the emotional ups and downs, as though it will instantly be the best thing that ever happened to us. Well, it eventually will be. But sometimes along the way there are negative emotions to deal with as well, particularly if you have many stubborn pounds to lose.

Over the years I have heard, read and witnessed hundreds of women's success stories with this program. Some tell incredible tales of 30 and 40 pounds lost in a matter of weeks. While those results are impressive, they are not the norm. The stories I've selected here aren't the most dramatic examples of weight loss, but they each come from differing perspectives: middle-age weight, emotional weight gain, insecurities, genetic weight, new-mother fat and eating disorders.

The stories in this chapter, including my own, are meant to help you understand that getting in shape is an emotional process as well as a physical chore. It's not always easy, but it's also not always hard. It will become a great source of pride, if you let it. Most importantly, I hope you realize that whatever emotions you confront in the process, the end result will be worth it. You must have faith that if you stick with this program, it will work for you as it has worked for me and many others.

Getting Fat, Just Like Everyone Else

*A*s I've already explained, I was one of those reed-thin youngsters. I worked out because it was a social thing, not so much because I needed to. I actually like to exercise, I like the people and I like the task. I love to set a personal best, like 50 manly push-ups.

In my thirties I began to put on weight, most of it right at the top of my thighs. This was my stubborn fat. It had been there, albeit less of it, when I barely weighed 100 pounds. It was there despite my varied exercise efforts. At just 5-foot-2, with nearly half my height in my torso, I have always been particularly conscious of my "stubby" legs.

When I was 39 I made a conscientious effort to get in the best shape of my life for the big 4-0! As my friends would say, I was not growing old graciously. I was angry at my age and I turned the throttle up full bore on my workouts.

At the time, I was in a relationship with a man who was quite adept at keeping me at arm's distance. You may know the type: the proverbial bachelor. Of course, I couldn't see it and went merrily about my life thinking that Saturday-night dating was a perfectly normal thing to do, forever. It left me with six evenings out of every week with nothing better to do than go to the health club. So I did.

Discovering Freestyle

It soon became apparent that working out six days a week was going to make me look like the Incredible Hulk. That's when I first began chang-

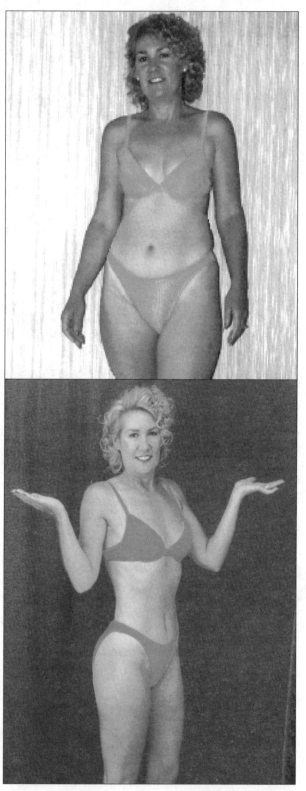

My weight loss took a total of ten months. Three months were wasted exercising wrong. Three months were spent rebuilding my base strength (level 1) and I dropped 25 pounds over the next four months.

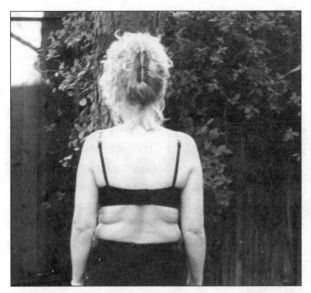

When I saw this photo I was shocked! Middle-age changed my fat storage patterns and my back had become absolutely flabby. This photo made me say 'enough is enough' and got me back in the gym.

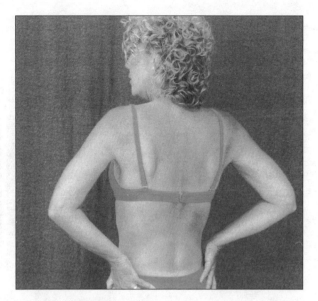

This photo was taken ten months later. Since this photo was taken, I've continued to work on the level three program and my back has become more toned and shapely than ever!

ing my workouts to de-emphasize muscle building. I began to use multiple-muscle exercises, some similar to the calisthenics I used to perform in high school. I did lots of pull-ups and push-ups. I even did military-style burpees and jumped rope. I did multiple sets of 25 to 30 lightweight squats. Some days I did sets of 50. I also roller-bladed 5 to 6 miles nearly every day. The end result was that my thigh bulges began to shrink, and I discovered the key principle behind Freestyle training: train the legs every day.

Although it took nearly a year, when I turned 40 I was indeed in the best shape of my life. However, I was also single and had come to realize I was in a dead-end relationship. My workouts were going well, but that was about the only good thing in my life.

My father was ill at the time, and since there was little else to keep me where I was, I decided to move to the city of Napa to be closer to him. Within weeks of the move I met my future husband, Chuck. Little did I know how much my life was about to change.

Cinderella After 40

I became a wife and stepmother almost overnight, and I'm here to tell you it was the toughest adjustment I've ever made. As though I had been living in some fantasy world, I had assumed being a stepmom would be like baby-sitting the kids for a weekend. Or maybe like the week Chuck, the kids and I spent together in Jamaica. Wrong.

I remember reading a book about stepparenting that first month and tossing it aside because it was so negative. It said to grin and bear it, because you're in a no-win situation. Six months later I understood what the book was talking about. The kids expected me to fix their meals, wash their clothes, drive them back and forth, buy them toys, play when they wanted to play and do hours of homework with them in the evenings. Basically, they expected me to be their mom. But when something went wrong, they didn't hesitate in letting me know I wasn't their mom. On Christmas and Mother's Day, I didn't receive any gifts. There weren't any "thank-yous," and the "I love yous" went to their birth mother, not me. It wasn't quite what I had expected.

The good news is that I survived that first year. By year two I had learned some parenting skills that have gone a long way in making the day-today "mom" tasks easier. I managed to make the transition from career woman to wife and step-mom, and now hardly blink at making two or three meals a day and picking up the inevitable toys and clothes lying around the house. I now also know much better what a stepparent's role is, and my expectations are far more realistic. Then there are the perks: last Mother's Day *I* got cards too.

However, during this two-year adjustment period I didn't work out. Sure, I made a visit now and then to the health club, but it wasn't much. In the back of my mind I somehow thought that I'd always be in shape; that fat was someone else's problem. I even remember telling Chuck when I met him, "What you see is what you get—if I'm not fat at 42, I don't think I'll ever be." Hah! Those words came back to bite me right in my big butt!

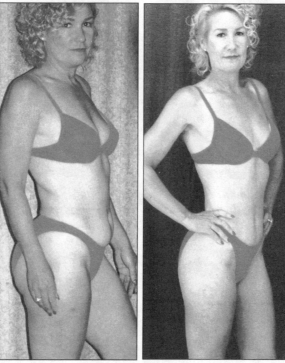

These photos were taken just five weeks apart, showing how dramatic the weight loss can be during the last part of level three when your body switches from fat-collecting to fat-burning.

Mine was a case of middle-age weight gain. I think I would have gained weight even if I had continued my workouts, though perhaps not as much.

The first thing I noticed was my lack of strength. Little tasks became tough. I bruised a rib water-skiing. I was listless during the day.

Then the weight crept on. The thigh bulges came back immediately, then the low-belly fat. I went from 118 to 128 pounds in the first year. Then my always-small waist began to disappear. Even my back got flabby. But the thing that irritated me most was my rear. It got huge. My bathrobe would get stuck in it when I stood up from a chair!

In the beginning, I was in denial. I continued to buy clothes one and two sizes too small. As I tried in vain to fasten the buttons in the changing room I'd tell myself "I'll lose the weight soon." Those clothes came home and sat in my closet with the tags still attached.

By age 45 things got worse. I was having hot flashes and I began experimenting with hormone therapy. I blamed the hormones for the weight gain that reached my all-time high of 140 pounds. I still carried a driver's license listing my weight at 100. What a joke!

Shame

I began wearing "fat people's clothes." The bigger and baggier the better. I was beginning to hate my body. Actually, hate is not a strong-enough word, I was repulsed by my body. I was so embarrassed about it that when Chuck "petted" my tummy one night I burst into tears. Right then I let him know that there were certain parts of my body I didn't want him to touch because of the shame I felt.

Finally, I said enough was enough. I was a pro at getting in shape; I knew what I had to do. So, to my husband's delight, I announced I was again going to give high priority to my workouts. I'd gotten this stepmother thing down, and now it was time to whip myself back into shape.

I whipped myself all right. Seven-day-a-week workouts; training the legs every day. Hours of cardio. Lunges until my knees ached. I did everything just as I'd done before, and nine weeks later I weighed 139 pounds and had lost barely an inch!

More than two months and nothing! It was devastating. I felt totally trapped by the body I was in.

There was no way an individual could possibly devote more energy to her workout. My diet was clean, for the most part. I seemed to be doing everything right, but nothing was working. I was now officially just like millions of American women: fat and unhappy. I had gained stubborn fat.

Fortunately, I know that diet and exercise will eventually win the battle and I'm not a quitter. There was something wrong with my former *Lower Body Solution*. It had worked before, and that's when I began to realize my program had worked on a younger body, and one that was in pretty good shape to begin with. My three-year layoff, plus my premenopausal age, had changed the parameters I had to work with.

I began to rethink the workout. I realized that middle-age fat was going to be tougher than any other fat I'd dealt with. I faced the reality that at middle age, when so many aspects of my professional and personal life had become easier, keeping weight off my body was going to be tougher than ever. I'd have to work harder and longer. I had to work smarter.

Supplementing Success

I made changes in my diet and added some key supplements. About an hour before my workouts I'd take two capsules of the amino acid L-Carnitine. Throughout the day I'd take six capsules of Pyruvex, a supplement that is formulated with special fat-burning agents. I purchase both from SportPharma (1-800-292-6536). I used (and still use) a meal replacement called Slim Again Weight Loss Shake from U.S. Nutriceuticals (1-877-292-6614) and during my workouts I have a fat-burner drink called Cutting Force by American Bodybuilding (1-800-627-0627). At night I took another amino acid, L-Glutamine (also from SportPharma), to help boost my lagging, middle-aged growth hormone production. I began to coordinate my exercise with my diet to maximize my own body's ability to burn fat and to recover after working out. I cut back and eased into the program, rebuilding my basic levels of strength and conditioning. In three weeks' time the program began to work, and I saw changes at last.

In three months' time the changes were noticeable. In six months' time I had transformed my body. Today, at 46, I can once again say that I'm getting into the best shape of my life. I now weigh 115 pounds, and plan to put on a little more muscle for tone and to drop about three more pounds to reach what I feel will be ideal proportions for my body type. I've even managed to get past a lot of those menopausal symptoms that were bugging me. Best of all, I've regained pride in my body and appearance. There aren't any "no touch" zones for my husband anymore, and I found lots of new clothes in my closet (tags still attached) that I fit into finally!

The experience has helped me fine-tune a program that works on tough weight—the old weight that has clung to our hips most of our lives; the stubborn weight that comes with middle age; the tenacious weight that seems impervious to diet and exercise.

Although the program was working extremely well for me, I wanted to be sure it would work for others. I began to work with heavier clients—one has more than 170 pounds to lose. I also began to work with older women—one in her 80s. While individual results vary, I'm pleased to announce that the program has successfully worked on everyone who has tried it!

Several of these women with *Lower Body Solution* success stories have been kind and generous enough to share their experiences with you. Sometimes it's tough to face the emotions of getting out of shape, and these women have graciously volunteered to share their sometimes painful stories to help you take up the cause and get on your own *Lower Body Solution* program. I thank them all.

New-Mother Fat

Throughout high school and her early 20s Becky McMaster never worried about her weight because she was naturally slim and active. Without much thought or effort, this 5-foot-8 brunette stayed in shape by doing the things she loved, like swimming and competitive ballroom dancing. But when she decided it was time for the pitter-patter of tiny feet, it spelled trouble for Becky's shapely figure. Big trouble.

Having her first baby proved much more difficult than she imagined. Sickness confined her to bed for the first six months and she packed on 50 pounds. By the time Becky gave birth to her first child at age 26 she was up to 200 pounds.

"I was very unhappy about what was happening to my body—I gained weight everywhere," Becky reveals. "My bellybutton popped out and

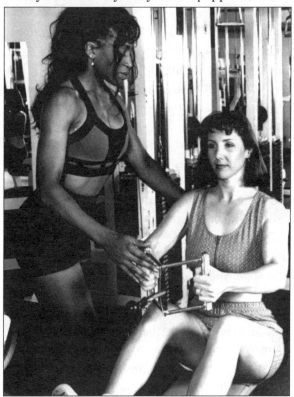

Becky's problem area was her waist and buttocks. On this program she slimmed her waist and toned up her rear.

my skin just felt tight all over. I was really concerned about stretch marks."

Post-Pregnancy Paunch

Becky did manage to lose about 30 pounds between the births of her first child and her second, and her weight hovered around 170 pounds. However, this was still a far cry from her prepregnancy weight of 135.

She had tried dieting, including the once-popular liquid diets that emerged in the late 1980s, but still the weight stuck.

"I had two cesarean sections, and as a result I have this stubborn paunch in my abdomen that was never there before," she laments.

Finally, she decided to get serious about her weight before it became impossible to control. A friend dragged her along to a weight training session with a personal trainer, urging her to "just check it out." Becky was leery of the gym—she had made a point of staying away from the "big burly muscle guys and cutesy girls in leotards" scene. But she reluctantly consented to give it a try. After one session she was hooked and got a personal trainer of her own.

"I had never lifted a weight in my life until October of 1996," Becky reveals. But by February of 1997, just five months later, her weight had dropped from 165 to 141—a strong testament to the fact that you can indeed lose weight through weight training!

After relocating to a new town and leaving her gym and her personal trainer behind, Becky regained some of her lost weight. Then she was referred to Tatiana Byrne, one of my stellar fitness trainers who is also featured in my *Lower Body Solution* aerobics video series. Tatiana was one of my first Freestyle-certified trainers, and she has worked with me in developing the program in this book. When Tatiana first met Becky, she knew she had met another candidate for our *Lower Body Solution*.

Tatiana began training her in February 1998 when Becky was flabby and weighed about 150 pounds. "My problem areas were my jiggly lower belly, inner thighs and the back of my arms—that attractive part that flaps around when you wave!"

In just four months on the *Lower Body Solution* program, Becky made some remarkable achievements. Although she lost only five pounds on the scale, Becky's body fat content measured at 18 percent, down from 28 percent before she started. "I definitely notice a difference in the way my body looks and feels. I look in the mirror now and see tone where I used to see flab! My rear end inal muscles that cannot be fully corrected through exercise. However, improvement is possible as other muscle fibers take over the tasks of those damaged in the surgeries.

Becky has improved her diet as well, although she confesses to having a weakness for cookies. "I drink a protein-and-veggie drink between meals to help take away my craving for cookies," she says. Instead of the two or three big meals a day she had been eating, Becky now eats five smaller meals throughout the day. She uses the Slim Again Weight Loss Shake in place of one or two meals a day and also the Slim Again Diet Bar. Most recently she's added Slim Again's Pyru-Lean pyruvate capsules. All three Slim Again products are available from U.S. Nutriceuticals 1-877-292-6614.

Tailored for a Busy Schedule

A busy full-time mom to four children—two stepchildren and two of her own—Becky's biggest problem is finding time to work out. "The only time I have right now is 1 1/2 hours two mornings a week when my youngest son is in preschool. Then I race to the gym for a workout. The greatest thing about the *Lower Body Solution* is that I still get results by doing it only two days a week!"

Becky's routine follows the Level Three workouts in this book, but Tatiana has combined the three mandatory days into two 1 1/2-hour sessions to better fit Becky's busy schedule.

On days away from the gym Becky stays active by walking and by caring for her high-energy kids. During summer she's an avid water-skier. She also uses some of the "thigh-blaster" home workouts from Chapter Seven. Although Becky doesn't have a big problem with fat on her thighs, she loves the extra lower-body strength and endurance.

"Living on a lake, we live for water-skiing and I ski at least once a day during the season," she says. "In the summer I practically live in a swimsuit, which makes me really self-conscious. But this year I am feeling better and looking firmer, and I have much more energy than I used to."

Becky is now just five pounds from her goal weight of 135 pounds. "I can do this!" she says.

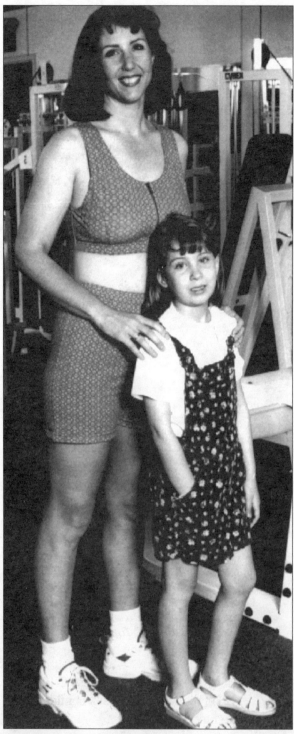

Becky, shown here with her daughter Sarah, is devoted to using the Lower Body Solution program not just to shed pounds, but as a "program for life."

used to be flat and shapeless; now I've got a butt!"

Becky's problem area remains her abdomen. The two C-sections caused damage to her abdom-

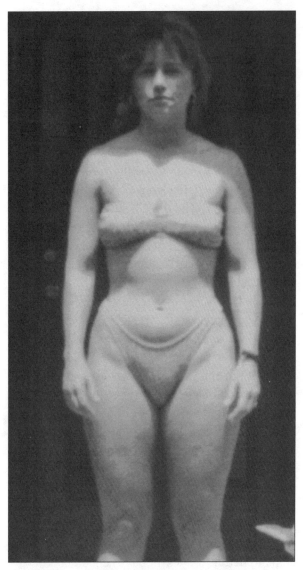

At her heaviest Kelly weighed 140 pounds, with most of the weight between her waist and her knees. She switched to high-frequency lower body exercise and the pounds began to melt.

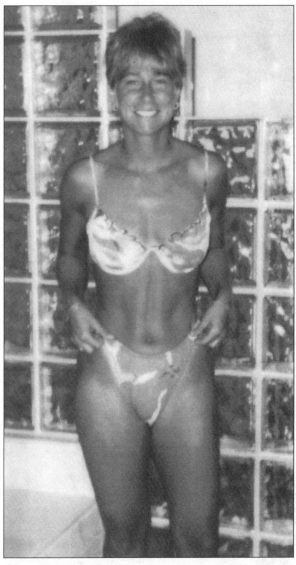

*Kelly slimmed down to 102 pounds. Now, four years later, she is a firm believer in the **Lower Body Solution** program and manages to maintain a slim and toned "hardbody" figure.*

Paring Down the "Pear" Shape

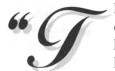here is no way that I could be doing what I'm doing today if I still had the weight," Kelly Bennett says from her Florida headquarters, where she masterminds the public relations and publicity for Extreme, a high-profile team of female fitness competitors. "I love what I do; I love working in the fitness field. But a few years ago I didn't have the self-confidence or the figure to be doing this."

Kelly has the classic "pear" shape. It's an inherited condition, but that doesn't make the situation feel any better. There is something very unsettling about disproportionate weight gain. Kelly remembers envying heavier women with even weight distribution. "They looked strong and athletic; I looked bulgy, awkward and out of shape." She recalls looking at her straight-on view in the mirror and almost wishing she could take a big butcher knife and slash off the offending hip swells.

As Kelly got chunkier her moods got darker. "Some days I was downright depressed," she says. "At one point I got down on my knees and prayed to God for the strength to lose weight and for a miracle to help me."

A Classic "Pear"

Nearly all of Kelly's weight accumulated in the area between her hips and her knees. At her heaviest, Kelly weighed 140 pounds. Some of you may think that sounds like a fine weight, but not if you're 27 years old and a diminutive 5-foot-3. Kelly knew it was just the beginning, and she feared that she'd soon look like the overweight Northerners who frequent the Florida beaches near her seaside home.

"Exercise wasn't my first line of defense; diet was," says Kelly, who claims to have tried every diet she could lay her hands on. "I was completely frustrated. I'd lose a few pounds, then gain it right back. I felt that my failure to lose weight was causing me to fail in other aspects of my life. I felt if I could only lose the weight, then everything would change for the better.

"I know that weight and appearance aren't everything. But for me it made such a difference in my self-confidence that my weight loss really did translate into success in other areas of my life."

Freestyle Transformation

Kelly's first success at controlling her weight began when someone handed her my *Freestyle Training* book. Soon, she was working in a Florida office distributing my books.

Kelly and I used to talk for hours on the phone about the program and both of our personal struggles to lose weight. "Your approach always made sense," says Kelly, who got so behind the Freestyle program that she says her friends nicknamed her "Miss Freestyle."

Kelly's enthusiasm transformed her body in

four months, chiseling the fat from her lower body. She got down to 102 pounds, and has managed to stay there for more than four years. Today, she has embraced the new *Lower Body Solution* workouts and recommends the system even for the "hardbodies" in Extreme.

"The exercise was a big part of the initial weight loss, but I've also made some changes in my diet that have helped keep the weight off," she says. "I was eating all the wrong foods for my body type. Pasta and bread were the two worst offenders. When I began to learn about glycemic indexes and started to cut out the carbs, I felt better. It's the first diet I've ever tried where I didn't feel like I was dieting."

Kelly likes the changes I've made to the exercise portion of the program. "Those lunges started bothering my knees, but the new program is something you can stick with, for life." She's been with the new program since the beginning, so I suppose I can nickname her "Miss Lower Body Solution" now.

Kelly, by the way, is now performing one-on-one diet and exercise consultation in the *Lower Body Solution*. She actually "visits" with you for a week, helping you fix meals at home, going grocery shopping, eating out and working out with you to help get your entire lifestyle on track for a whole-body solution. She comes with excellent references and can be reached through our offices at (707) 257-2348.

Progress, Not Perfection

Several months ago, on the way to the gym, Deborah Ryan turned to me with what was obviously a very difficult and emotional issue she needed to discuss.

"Laura," she announced, "I don't want to be the fat girl in your book."

Tears welled up in her eyes and spilled down her face. She then recounted her life story—a battle with weight, food, addictions and depression. "It's too much pressure for me at this point. I'm afraid that looking at a picture of myself in your book, feeling ugly and overweight, will only undermine my efforts to get the weight off."

"Okay," I said. Getting the weight off Deborah was far more important than another before-and-after photo for the book. I wasn't going to push the subject; I just let her talk.

She said through her tears that I couldn't understand the emotional pain of being truly fat. "To be a large woman in a supposed-to-be-thin world has been, at times, a hell for me." I listened and I continued training Deborah; I still do, as a matter of fact. And she's right. I don't understand what it's like to be a person trying to lose more than 75 pounds. I don't know what it feels like to be really fat.

Fighting An Eating Disorder

Deborah hasn't had the world presented to her on a silver platter. At age four a tragic car accident changed her life. She spent her fifth birthday in the hospital undergoing facial reconstructive surgery that helped her but didn't completely correct the extensive damage. Today, due to nerve damage, she has partial paralysis on one side of her face that yields a crooked smile. She has spent her life adjusting and coping with this disfigurement and still wonders what her life would have been like had that car not collided with that little girl so many years ago.

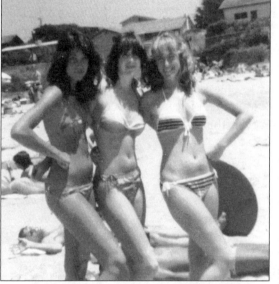

Deborah, far left, weighed just 135 in high school. The weight crept on over a period of ten years. Her goal is to slim down to 155 pounds.

"From my earliest memory I felt different and 'less than' others," she says. "I was teased relentlessly—kids can be very cruel. That really set the stage for me feeling extremely self-conscious about my face and body."

A chubby child, Deborah turned to food to soothe her feelings of anger, low self-esteem and

depression. Sneaking food and binge eating became regular patterns in her life throughout elementary and high school. "Often the only things I looked forward to during the day were mealtimes and snacking."

Deborah finished high school with good grades and moved on to college with plenty of friends. Like most college students, she partied. However, drinking soon began to take on an exhilarating and increasingly more important role in her life. "When I took a drink of alcohol, for the first time in my life I felt freedom from my self-consciousness. I felt freedom from my fear of people and what they thought of me—the fears that had been driving me my whole life. I honestly thought alcohol was the answer to all my problems; I had found the magic elixir!"

After college came a good career move working for a magazine—quick advancement and the pressure to succeed. To cope, Deborah repeatedly turned to food and alcohol for ease and comfort, and she began to pack on the pounds at an alarming rate. This started a series of diets and bingeing which threw her metabolism into a tailspin. "When I could manage to get some weight off with starvation diets and pills, it would all come back again, and then some, as soon as I went off the diet. Plus, my obsession for food was steadily progressing and I no longer reacted sanely or reasonably toward food. In the last eight years of on-and-off-again dieting I had gained more than 50 pounds!"

Hitting Rock Bottom

Advancement to a high-paying job as technical writer for an aerospace company brought more pressures, and for a while food took a back seat to alcohol. This time she slowly hit rock bottom.

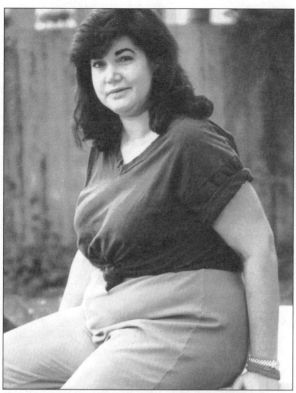

This was Deborah on Day 1 of the **Lower Body Solution** *program weighing her all-time high of 230 pounds.*

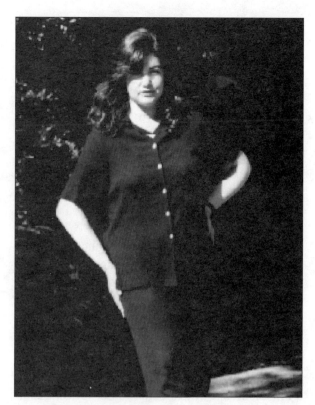

This was Deborah five months later and 25 pounds lighter. Her motto is: "Progress not perfection."

At home bottles of wine and vodka started disappearing fast. And, just as with food, Deborah began sneaking drinks so no one would know how much she was drinking. "I had this hole inside me of loneliness, shame, and unworthiness. If I did manage to fool people by looking okay on the outside, inside I was a nervous, despairing wreck."

On the verge of losing her job, she joined Alcoholics Anonymous. "With alcohol out of my system my life definitely has improved, but I still battle with food. I am a compulsive overeater and, just like alcohol, it is an addiction for me. The difference is I don't have the option of eliminating food from my life."

No More Quick Fixes

Now in her thirties, Deborah has taken time to do some soul-searching and has devoted many years to "fixing the much bigger things in life that really matter." One of those things is her physical health. When she came to me her weight had hit an all-time high of 230 pounds, which put her at high risk for many obesity-related disorders.

At 5-foot-10, Deborah is a big woman. In college, running two miles a day on the beach, she got down to 140 pounds, which she says was almost too light for her. At between 150 and 160 pounds she'll look great, but she's no longer deluding herself with any "quick-fix" ideas. "I know that I'm in this for the long haul. I didn't get this way overnight, so it's going to take a while to get out of it; maybe even years. But, that's okay because today I am making peace with my mind, my body and my relationship with food."

Her journey with the *Lower Body Solution* has not been easy, but it is working. Years of dieting and bingeing have packed some very serious and stubborn weight on her.

Emphasis on Exercise, Not Diet

"Right now I just don't feel capable of dieting," she has said. Still, I've been quite proud of the changes she has made. She rarely goes to fast-food places. She has slowly traded high-fat foods for the low- and reduced-fat varieties and even leaves food on her plate at restaurants. At my urging she is now also using L-Glutamine (SportPharma 1-800-292-6536) before bed to decrease her sugar cravings and increase her growth hormone production for better metabolism. "I am trying to listen to my body's signals of hunger and satiation. These signals have been warped for so long, but I'm starting to notice them again."

While all these changes are positive, Deborah has still not made a significant reduction in the calories she's eating. What she has done is made a major commitment to exercise.

A Real Commitment

"This is the first real commitment I've ever made to exercise in my life. When I started, I was so weak. I also expected to lose 25 pounds in just a few months, but I've come to accept that isn't the way it happens. I have definitely noticed changes in my body in the four months that I have been exercising. I can see and feel my muscles getting toned—muscles I never knew I had! I have more energy and I sleep better. And one of the best benefits is the effect on my mental health. My depression has lessened and my whole attitude toward life has changed.

"I never thought I would enjoy a workout. I just thought of exercise as something to be endured. Plus, I was intimidated by all those big, complicated-looking machines at the gym. Now, most days I actually look forward to going to the gym. I have made peace with weights and those daunting machines. In fact, I have found that I like lifting weights because I can see the improvements I am making very clearly."

Deborah is losing two to four pounds a month. I expect that rate will improve as she gets further into the program. She began as a complete newcomer to weight training, following the level one program in this book. She is now much stronger and each week reaches new benchmarks in stamina and strength.

"It's been about three years since I've owned a

swimsuit," she said recently. "This year I'm going to buy one and think about wearing it." Deborah's motto for other women in her shoes: "Progress, not perfection."

Fighting Genetics

As a Samoan woman, Marama Smith is genetically predisposed to have a big form, especially chunky legs and thighs. But, looking at her petite size 5 figure now you would never guess she inherited those genes. In fact, Marama says that people often don't believe her when she reveals her nationality—proof that the "large Samoan" stereotype has a tight hold on our mindsets.

Growing up, Marama had pretty much accepted her "chunkiness" and didn't do much to fight her body type. In high school Marama was anything but athletic. She was an inactive couch potato with a preference for fast food and a cigarette habit to boot. At 5-foot-3, she weighed a very solid 140 pounds.

Bulking Up With The Guys

When she turned 20 a job listing caught her eye—it was a recruitment ad for firefighters. From that day forward it was Marama's dream to become a woman firefighter. However, she says she almost failed the academy because she was so out of shape.

"That was when I realized that if this was the career I really wanted, I had to get myself in shape," she says. "I didn't want to fail at this. I had heard all the rumors that some men thought women couldn't pull their weight as firefighters—that just motivated me to work harder! I felt like I had to prove myself."

Prove herself she did. Marama came on strong and pulled through her academy training displaying as much skill and strength as her male classmates.

How did she do it? By heading straight for the gym, to those stacks of weights and machines that her male contemporaries were training with. And then she set about training hard, like a bodybuilder, following the lead of other buffed and strong firemen.

As expected, with her determination and dedication Marama saw results quickly and she was getting strong and fit. But, she was also getting quite muscular—just like the guys—and bulking up her already thick legs.

"I didn't know there was any other way to train," she says. "But, now I know I wasn't lifting weights smart, just hard. I wasn't satisfied with my body and I was also injuring myself from time to time."

So what happened? What changed? Marama was spotted at the gym one day by certified *Lower Body Solution* personal trainer Tatiana Byrne. Tatiana knew instantly that the program would

work for Marama and approached her. Marama was skeptical at first—the results she promised just seemed too good to be true!—but she was willing to give it a try because of Tatiana's excellent reputation. Within two weeks Marama noticed a difference.

Shape-Shifter

"I never saw my body shape change so fast!" she says. "I never thought lifting light weights would work. But, with the right tempo and number of reps, it really does! Also, I had never worked out five and six days a week before—that really sped up my results."

The supercharged combination of weights and cardio training performed five times a week was the key to changing Marama's metabolism, which in turn began to melt the pounds off

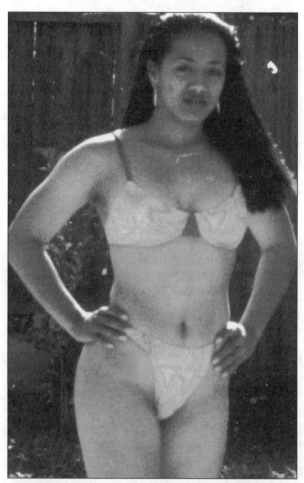

At the start of her Lower Body Solution *program Marama was "chunky." She believed her "thick" figure was the fate of genetics.*

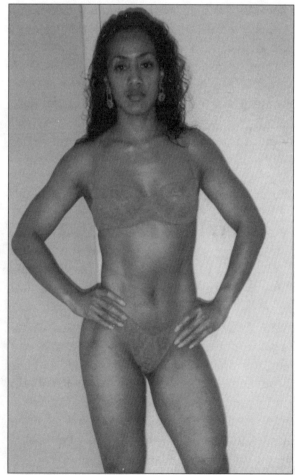

After just six weeks on the Lower Body Solution *Marama's figure had almost completely transformed from chunky to slim.*

rapidly. At one point, just a few months into her *Lower Body Solution* training, Marama told Tatiana, "Lighten up, I'm losing weight and inches too fast!"

The dramatic changes Marama experienced are not the exception on this program but more often the rule. Her bulkiness gave way to softer, smoother, more feminine lines. As she puts it, she "leaned out."

In addition to modifying her training, Marama decided that she was going to "eat clean" and avoided fast food, junk food and red meat. She ate chicken, fish, fruits and vegetables in six small meals per day. This combination of diet and *Lower Body Solution* exercise worked, and Marama has maintained her weight loss and a shapely 125-pound hourglass figure with a mere 12 percent body fat for more than a year. Equally important, Marama is in top condition and strong enough to meet the rigors of her demanding, male-dominated career as a firefighter.

"I am breaking all the barriers for my race," Marama says, "because genetically we are big! People who meet me now think I'm this size because I've been an athlete all my life. No, I tell them, far from it! I owe it all to my personal trainer and the *Lower Body Solution*!"

Starving for Acceptance

Today at age 53, Patty Atkinson is in the best shape of her life, feeling strong and confident about her body. Standing 5-foot-6, she's a svelte 110 pounds. But it hasn't been an easy road to get to where she is. Overweight as a child and teen, Patty has waged a war against flab and has fought mightily—perhaps too hard—to maintain a vital, youthful appearance her entire adult life.

In a room full of people Patty garners admiring glances from men half her age. But she remembers a time when admirers were few and far between—a painful time in those already rocky teenage years when she was fat and miserable and felt helpless to change her situation.

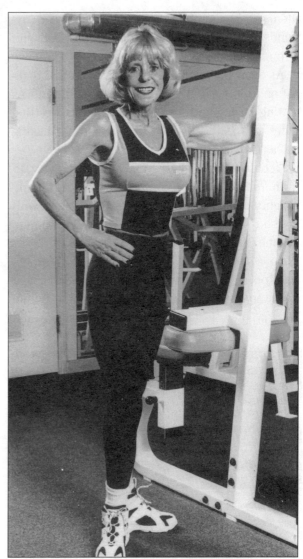

Pressure to be thin has plagued Patty her entire life. Today, at 53, she has developed a new and healthier attitude about her body and owes much of that to her new **Lower Body Solution** *exercise program.*

Pressured to Be Thin

At her heaviest Patty weighed 165 pounds, which, while not obese, was awkward and chunky on her small-boned frame. Patty's weight seriously affected the way she felt about herself. This set the stage for a lifelong struggle with low self-esteem and a pervasive feeling of not fitting in with others. And growing up in a house full of thin people only made matters worse.

"My mother was constantly putting me on diets," says Patty. "I tried everything, including crash diets and diet pills, which only made me feel sick and shaky." And still the weight stayed on.

"I remember what a nightmare it was to go clothes shopping," she reveals. "While my sisters could zip through the racks and find what they wanted, I was stuck wearing big, ugly, shapeless things. I got teased in school about it."

To compensate for her appearance, Patty became the class clown. In her sophomore year of high school she was even voted "wittiest" in her class. Still, although she had plenty of friends, she didn't like herself. "I hid behind humor. Everyone saw a happy, cheerful face, but inside I was sad and hurting. I desperately wanted to be thin.

"I always hung out with the guys, but they didn't notice me the way I wanted them to notice me. To them I was just the 'cute fat girl.' To this day I hate being called 'cute' because it reminds me of those days."

Her diet consisted largely of foods we thought were good for us back then, like lots of high-fat dairy products and red meat. Plus, in Patty's family the rule was you had to finish eating everything on your plate (sound familiar?). If she complained or questioned why, the answer was something about "children starving in China."

Something Clicked

The turning point in Patty's battle with weight came during her junior year in high school. "I got to the point where I was sick and tired of being depressed. Something inside me just clicked and I got motivated to do whatever it took to get the weight off. I believe I got to a place in my life where I was mentally ready—and mature enough—to follow through with it."

Patty immediately cut out all junk food and increased her exercise. Since she had always been somewhat of a tomboy, getting daily exercise by swimming, biking and other sports was the easiest part of her plan. Food was another story.

"I lost weight pretty quickly, she says, "but not without feeling hunger pains all the time. Cutting down on the portions of food I ate was really tough for me."

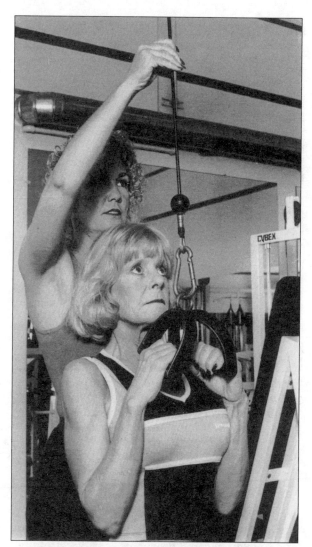

Patty still struggles with the idea that a little weight gain is okay. But her energy and enthusiasm in the gym are paying off with new muscle tone, strength and self-confidence.

To Patty, enduring some hunger was not nearly as bad as how she had felt being fat. Once the weight came off, all of a sudden those boys who hadn't noticed her before began to ask her out. "I loved every minute of it! I only wondered why I hadn't done it sooner!"

The more weight she lost the more popular she became. And that feeling of acceptance—the feeling she had longed for her whole life—fueled her motivation to diet harder, even when her friends were regularly enjoying burgers and fries. Her preoccupation with her weight was starting to take on a life of its own.

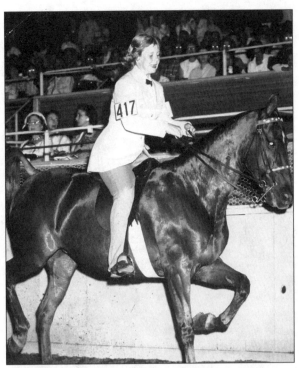

*Patty's obsession with being thin began in high school when she was "chubby," as compared to her mother and sisters. A better self-image has been one of the biggest benefits to come from her **Lower Body Solution** program.*

Compulsive Undereater

Patty was married straight out of high school and quickly became pregnant. Fear of getting fat again plagued her, but she vowed not to give in. She became a compulsive undereater. Incredibly, Patty's average weight gain for each of her five pregnancies was only 10 to 20 pounds, and although her doctors were concerned, she gave birth to five healthy kids (all girls!).

In addition to her near-starvation diets, Patty was also going overboard on exercise—anything that would burn calories and keep off fat. "I started doing sit-ups the day I got home from the hospital," she says. "I did hundreds of sit-ups all the time."

After her last pregnancy at age 30, Patty's weight hovered around 125 to 130 pounds. Triumph! she thought—she had made it through a period of life when many women pack on pounds that stay with them for life.

Mid-Life Crises

In her mid and late 40s her feelings of triumph began to wane with new changes in her body. "My skin was losing its tone. I was flabby. I felt like I was losing my body to old age. In the past I could diet myself back into shape, but I knew diet wasn't going to help my deterioration now."

Determined to fight back, she joined a gym. However, she felt frustrated because the trainers "babied" her. "Because of my age, they didn't push me. They led me to believe that this was the best my body could be and that I just had to deal with it. That depressed me even more, but I just accepted the advice."

Patty continued to restrict her calories and to weight train, but the results were never personally satisfying. Then, at age 52, a bomb was dropped into Patty's life that would change things forever.

After 34 years of marriage, Patty returned from a week-long visit with one of her daughters to find a "Dear John" note on the kitchen counter and divorce papers in the mail—her husband had left her for a woman 20 years younger. "I was devastated. I felt numb and was unable to eat, sleep or think rationally for months—depression set in big time."

It was this crisis that got Patty to seriously look at many aspects of her life and behavior. Her body had been a source of pride. It was also a source of hard work and sacrifice. In many ways, so was her marriage. But in the case of her body, Patty had a chance to regain the pride.

Searching for a new approach to her fitness, and a place to hide as the divorce proceeded, Patty found a new personal trainer—one who told her that yes (!!), she could improve her body at her age. "Finally, someone told me there was hope, that I didn't have to give up just because I had reached middle age!"

It was at this same time that a friend gave her a copy of my first book, *Freestyle Training*, and then introduced us. She decided to give *Freestyle* a try. It can't hurt, she thought. So, twice a week she worked with her new personal trainer, who motivated and encouraged her, and on other days she did the Freestyle routines on her own. As the *Lower*

Body Solution program began to take shape, Patty became more interested and began to use the new routines with renewed ambition and vigor. Soon she felt the veil of depression lifting.

Not Just About Losing Weight

"Getting in shape and following a program as comprehensive as the *Lower Body Solution* wasn't really about losing weight, not for me," says Patty. "At the time I was so depressed that I needed to do something to make myself feel better. I definitely needed toning up—especially my problem area, my butt, hips and thighs—but I did it just as much to vent my anger and anxiety at the gym."

To help build up her flagging muscle tone Patty also changed her near-starvation-influenced diet tactics. She began eating four to five small meals a day with lots of protein. I also got her hooked on the Slim Again trio of products from U.S. Nutriceuticals (1-877-292-6614) that consists of an antioxidant anti-aging vitamin formula, a meal replacement drink and a nutrition bar for when those sugar cravings hit . "In addition to the supplements, my diet now consists of fruit, vegetables and skinless chicken breasts.

"I don't really have to worry about calories very much today, but I still watch them. My weight was such a traumatic issue for me when I was young that I still think I could go back there if I let things slip. I rarely weigh myself, but I can feel it if I gain two or three pounds. If I ate French fries every day I could be huge. I don't know that for sure, but I don't want to find out!"

The Right Stuff

This threefold program of a new diet and supplements, *Lower Body Solution* exercises and a personal trainer to keep her motivated has yielded big results for Patty. Her muscles are now noticeably more toned, firm and well defined. Her skin looks tighter; her energy is up. "I can't believe how quickly it happened. I actually have shape to my legs now and I love wearing shorts again!"

In other words, Patty is proud of her body again. And she's proud of it for all the positive energy and work she has put in—not for the sacrifice and deprivation of starvation diets.

Being suddenly single at this stage in her life was not something Patty ever envisioned, but each day she builds a little more self-esteem and a little more confidence. Having sacrificed many of her wants—and gladly so—for the sake of her husband and children, Patty now has a whole world of options available to her. For the first time she's discovering who she is and what she wants out of life.

"I could be an embittered 'man-hater' because of the divorce, but I'm not. I like men. What I know now is that I don't need a man to validate me or make me happy. Don't get me wrong, I am not always happy with myself—I still have days when I feel fat, ugly and depressed—but that's normal. There is life after divorce!

"There's no doubt it gets harder to stay in shape as you get older; it has been that way with me. But it's never too late to start. I see so many old people who just lie around all the time and struggle even to walk. I'm not leaving this world in bed; I'm going out kicking!"

Success is what this book is all about. Your own story will be added to these success stories soon, I'm sure. While the situations and goals of each of these women is varied, they all have one thing in common: the *Lower Body Solution*. Each has used the program to accomplish their goals. If you've read closely, you may have noticed that some individuals have slightly modified the program to their needs.

The *Lower Body Solution* program is written so that it can be modified easily. Each of the workouts (in level three) are designed so that you can work out anywhere from two to six days a week, depending on your available time. You may recall that Becky McMaster's personal trainer modified the three-day-per-week routine to two longer sessions. Flexibility is key in this program. You can even miss a week or two, and still get right back on the program!

Personally, I made a few modifications to the program. I followed level one exactly as written in order to rebuild my base level of strength. I also followed level two exactly as written in order to prime myself for the high-frequency workouts in level three.

Once I began level three I made a few modifications. I relied frequently on the home workouts in Chapter Seven in order to maintain a five- and six-day-per-week schedule throughout the nine weeks. I also added ten to fifteen minutes to the cardio portions of the routines beginning in week four, and used the interval sessions described in Chapter Six whenever possible. I believe these modifications, plus my supplement regimens, were what helped me to achieve the dramatic fat loss during my last five weeks of the program.

I continue to work at sculpting my best-ever figure by working through the level three program.

However, I now do the routine four or five days a week and I stick to the cardio portions exactly as written. My weight remains under control, a condition I hope to maintain for the rest of my life.

Exercise is absolutely key to weight loss, particularly for loss of stubborn fat such as middle-age fat and fat that is genetically pre-programmed. However, when it comes to weight loss, exercise shares the stage with diet. Each of the women in this book achieved success on the *Lower Body Solution* exercise program; however, their diet programs differed greatly. In Chapter Fifteen I discuss several diet approaches. I believe that effective eating is achieved once you've found the foods and eating patterns that can promote weight loss without a struggle or feelings of deprivation. Finding the proper diet regimen will take time, and probably some trial and error. For this reason I suggest you keep an open mind regarding diets, and try them all.

While I was losing weight, many people asked what my secret was. "It's not a secret, it's my *Lower Body Solution*," I'd say. Nine times out of ten the person would give me an elbow nudge and a wink, and say "Come on, what are you *really* doing?"

The truth is that I really do use the *Lower Body Solution*! However, I also take certain supplements that I believe have been very beneficial to my weight loss efforts. While I am not a paid endorser of any of these products, to be perfectly forthright I feel I must mention all of the products I use by name. To be helpful, I have also provided phone numbers for these products whenever possible.

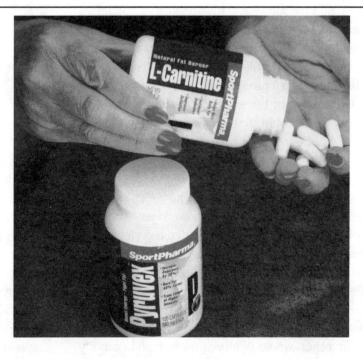

Why Women Get Fat

*I*f we have a *Lower Body Solution*, there must be a lower body problem. Most women at this point can roll their eyes like my 14-year-old stepdaughter and say, "Duh!"

The lower body—in particular, the hips, thighs, buttocks and low belly—is the area where most women store fat. Some women are so genetically programmed for this condition that their upper bodies look as though they were detached at the waist and placed on top of some fat alien's lower body. Further, even when weight loss is achieved, the last place most women lose weight is in the lower body.

Although the lower body is a big problem for many women, this book could have also been called the *Total Body Solution* because it will lower your overall body fat. However, the beauty of the program is that it will attack that stubborn fat that makes most women's lives miserable, the lower-body fat.

Will it work for men? Probably not. The *Lower Body Solution* is written entirely for women. You can forget the "one size fits all" approach to exercise. This is a program specifically tailored for women only.

The *Lower Body Solution* is designed to burn fat, a lot of fat and really stubborn fat. Why all the attention to fat? Because genetically, fat is natural on a female body.

How do women slim down? The Lower Body Solution!

The Difference Between Men and Women

Anyone can get fat, and most certainly, men do. As a matter of fact, men can get real fat, with guts that prodigiously spill over their most manly parts and render those family jewels inaccessible. The "beer belly" is a male problem; fat in the lower body and belly is a female problem. While both types of fat are the same, our society somehow deems fat on a woman less desirable than fat on a man. This makes a woman's fight against fat more personal than it is for most men.

For example, I have a girlfriend who smokes. As I pleaded with her to consider the health ramifications, she finally confessed to me that she had tried quitting once and in the process gained more than 70 pounds.

"I know people can be cruel and rude about my smoking," she told me. "But that's nothing compared to how cruel the world can be when you're fat. I've gone to doctors and they've pointed out that I come from a family of

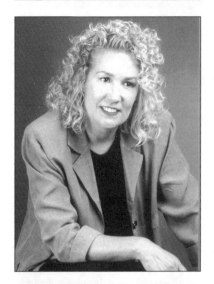

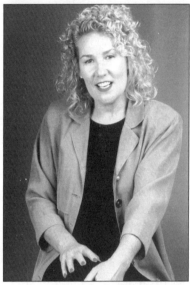

It never fails to amaze me that so many people have trouble understanding that the bodies of men and women are different, and therefore require different programs, protocols and exercises. If you learn nothing else from this book, please remember to steer clear of exercise and diet solutions that are unisex in their approach. If you train and eat like a man, you'll look like one!

obese women. Fat is in my genes.

"The nicotine is the only thing keeping me slim, and I'd rather be skinny and dead than fat and alive."

Unbelievable, isn't it? The sad thing is, I understand how she felt.

Women and men do not just think differently about fat; they actually gain, store and lose it differently. For a man, 15 percent body fat is considered normal. For a woman, 23 percent is normal. That's just a fact of life.

The differences in how we lose fat are never more apparent than when a couple tries to go on a diet together—something I don't advise women to do. Weight can literally fall off a man with seemingly little effort, while it fights a hearty battle to continue clinging to a woman's thighs even though she deprives herself more than the man and exercises harder!

One of the differences between men and women is that women have more fat-storage enzymes than men. The reason for this rather cruel trick of nature is that fat is necessary for regular estrogen production, which in turn is necessary for women to conceive and give birth. Unfortunately, it also makes weight gain easier for women than for men.

Why Fat Is More Stubborn Than Ever

In *Outsmarting the Female Fat Cell*, Debra Waterhouse, M.P.H., R.D., points out that one of the problems women have with dieting is that low-calorie diets actually increase the number of fat-storing enzymes. Ever skipped meals or eaten salads to cut down on calories? Of course! Almost every woman in America over the age of 25 has been on a low-calorie diet at some point in her life.

According to Waterhouse's book, research done at Cedars-Sinai Medical Center and other institutions found that diets that are too low in calories can double the number of fat-storing enzymes. This explains why women fall victim to the Yo-Yo Diet Syndrome: low-calorie diets increase the fat-storage abilities, so once a diet is abandoned and the dieter begins eating regularly, her body quickly regains the weight, and more!

At the heart of our struggle with our weight is the fact that fat is what keeps our estrogen stores high so that we can conceive and have babies. It's what allows us to feed those babies. If fat levels fall too low a woman will stop having menstrual periods and may become infertile, a condition known as amenorrhea.

Several centuries ago, when famines were still a common occurrence, a woman's generous fat stores ensured that she would be able to procreate despite lean times. That was a very good thing a few centuries ago—today, it stinks.

Another reason women struggle so desperately with fat is that we have low lean body mass (muscle) and therefore slow metabolisms.

Too much aerobic exercise will decrease our lean muscle mass even more. Therefore, as with a low-calorie diet, by performing aerobics to lose weight you can actually set your body up to gain even more fat than you would if you didn't exercise at all!

As we age our percentage of lean body mass decreases, slowing our metabolisms even more. When this combines with a less active lifestyle, fat is the inevitable result. Then whoa! When menopause comes along our bodies again go into a fat-preservation mode in a futile attempt to keep its estrogen levels intact. The end result is that even though you weren't born fat, chances are good that you will eventually become fat.

How This Book Can Change Your Life

For those of you who have read my book *Freestyle Training*, the *Lower Body Solution* is an extension of that program. It's Freestyle, and a whole lot more. It's what you do after you've tried Freestyle. It's what you do if Freestyle wasn't the solution to your problem. It's Freestyle for everybody, not just the hardbodies.

When you hire a personal trainer there are two things that individual brings you that have been proven to get results. One is motivation. The other is variety. This book is meant to be your personal trainer. It's meant to motivate you, and there's enough variety built in to keep you excited about each week's workouts and to also keep producing the changes you want to see.

By following the routines week-by-week exactly as written, you will become healthier, stronger and slimmer. For women with truly stubborn fat, there is an arsenal of stubborn fat-fighters built into the program. Depending on your circumstances, you can turn up the heat with additional fat-burning techniques to get the results you're working toward. This program doesn't assume you're going to lose fat easily. It assumes you've got stubborn fat and it touches upon every possible diet and exercise technique available for you to lose it!

Paring Down the Pear Shape

Fat is lost from different areas of the body at different rates. It tends to be lost first from the last place it was gained. This is why a woman with a lifelong problem of storing fat in the lower body will have a long battle to lose fat from this area.

While it is impossible to target a specific body part for fat loss, it is possible to waste away some of the muscle girth in a particular area. This is a phenomenon Coach Kim Goss first discovered while working with figure skaters, and is part of what formed our 1994 thesis on weight training for weight loss.

A big problem with female figure skaters is they must have a high degree of muscle strength in order to perform the jumps, yet they need to be physically small and petite for aesthetic appeal. Even

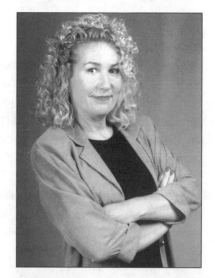

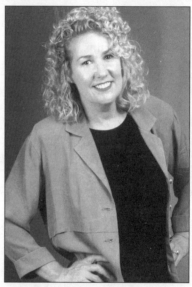

Freestyle Training *attracted a loyal and dedicated following. This new program encompasses many of the same principles, but with a more universal approach. My goal with this program is to help all women, no matter what age or size, to achieve the best body possible. It's worked for me, and if you give it a chance, it will work for you too.*

before Tonya Harding became involved with the bashing of Nancy Kerrigan's knee, she was already criticized by much of the skating community because of her large, muscular thighs.

One of Coach Goss's early successes was with figure skater Karen Carpenter. At five-foot-two, Karen weighed 148 pounds and was nicknamed "Freight Train" by her peers. Coach Goss put her on a program of medium-intensity leg exercises performed five days a week. This high-frequency training actually caused the size of Karen's thighs to reduce while helping her burn more calories for overall weight loss. The program included a daily transition of exercises in order not to overtrain or injure the legs. The result was that Karen slimmed down to a nicely proportioned 104 pounds, and she has maintained her figure ever since with minimal effort.

The *Lower Body Solution* will utilize this same high-frequency approach to reduce your lower body areas. But there is much more to it than training the legs every day. As I've learned since writing *Freestyle Training*, the exercises performed each day must be carefully planned. Too much repetition, such as performing the same aerobic routine or the same set of lunges every day, can result in overuse injuries and stagnated results. To be effective the program must always progress through varying cycles of exercises and intensities. Proper tempo and rest intervals also must be adhered to. After more than three years of testing, evaluation, reworking and documenting countless success stories, the *Lower Body Solution* spells out for you a clear-cut, precise plan for reducing even the most difficult spots on your body.

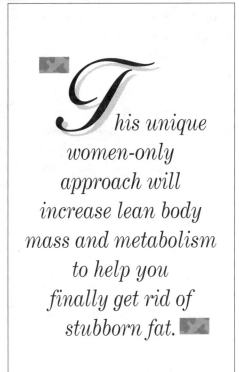

This unique women-only approach will increase lean body mass and metabolism to help you finally get rid of stubborn fat.

Muscle Versus Fat

The exercise program in the *Lower Body Solution* is so precise because it treads a very fine line. Muscle tone and lean body mass are desirable; big muscle is not. Remember, the reason men have an easier time controlling their bodyweight is that they generally have more lean body mass. Lean body mass requires more energy to sustain. A pound of blubber basically just sits there, but a pound of muscle is metabolically buzzing and burning calories even while it's at rest.

Aerobics form a part of the *Lower Body Solution*, but the program primarily relies on weight training. Intense aerobics will certainly burn off most of your body fat, but it will also eat up your lean body mass, making your skin appear to hang off your body like the skin on a Sharpei puppy. It's not a healthy condition and, especially in a swimsuit, it's not attractive.

The *Lower Body Solution* follows a weight training program designed for women, one that will promote 1) lean body mass, 2) an increase in metabolic rate, and 3) an increase in natural growth hormone production. This trio is the magic behind the program, along with the fact that the weight training routines are designed positively not to build excessively large muscle size.

For some of you, that part about stimulating production of growth hormone may sound alarming. I know that's a scary-sounding hormone, but it is present in all of us. Growth hormone levels are highest when we are young and growing. As we age, growth hormone production decreases considerably. This is one of the reasons it becomes harder to lose fat as we age—the abundant growth hormone of our youth helps maintain lean muscle mass to keep those metabolisms up. There has been a recent trend by "rejuvenation clinics" to provide growth hormone, at a hefty price, to restore some of the vigor and muscle tone of our youth. I don't advocate women using growth hormone supplementation because the long-term side effects are unknown, but stimulating growth hormone production naturally is a great way to help you get your weight under control. The pace of the exercise in this program helps to accomplish that.

As we consider the many reasons why women get fat, let's not forget the fact that American society has only recently decided that rail-thin is good. Just take a look at Marilyn Monroe, Jane Mansfield or even Elizabeth Taylor in their sex-kitten years and you'll be aghast at how "fat" these women were. Sexy? Very. But in a different era.

Today's supermodels are not typical women. Most are freaks of nature with incredibly wonderful bone structure and oddball metabolisms that let them stay well below normal body fat levels while not exercising and eating anything they please.

Striving for perfection is one thing, but striving for the unattainable—which is what the supermodels embody—is unrealistic and unhealthy.

It's important to be realistic about what you can ultimately accomplish with your body. You may never be as thin as you were in your teenage years, and most certainly, never as slim as the supermodels. Also bear in mind that too thin isn't sexy, it's sick. All too many times I've watched morbidly underweight women come to the health club and put in two hours on the stairclimber or treadmill. The supermodel image is to blame for why some women simply think they are fat. Still others are fat because they realize the impossibility of attaining this ideal, so they give up trying to improve their shape.

The *Lower Body Solution* can't make you tall if you're short and it can't make you small-boned if you weren't born that way. It can help you control your weight, even if it's been out of control your entire life. It can shrink your hips and thighs, even if they're disproportionately big. It can get you in the best shape of your life, for the rest of your life.

Are You Healthy?

There's no question that society's idolization of stick-thin women has messed with our collective mindset when it comes to our bodies and fat. Even though our intellect tells us that six percent body fat is sickly, in our hearts we still believe we can never be too rich or too thin. Thank goodness science has given us some objective measurements to check on our body fat and health.

Body Mass Index

Assessments have come a long way since I was a kid and we relied on the height-weight chart on the doctor's wall. Of the many means of establishing "healthy" weight today, the best is a combination of the Body Mass Index (BMI), the hip-to-waist ratio and a simple lifestyle checklist.

For those unfamiliar with it, BMI provides a measure of our body's ratio of fat-to-lean muscle mass. This index is considered superior to others in that it allows for some individuals who may weigh heavy on a height-weight chart, but who are carrying more muscle than fat. Although it's an improvement, I feel a more accurate gauge of health requires all three measurements.

The point to remember is that fat isn't just unattractive, it can kill us. Being seriously overweight greatly increases your risk of diabetes, hypertension and other chronic disorders that, even if they don't kill you, can drastically reduce the quality of your life.

Here is my three-part test for measuring your health risk.

1.
. First, calculate your BMI:

I have seen several ways to calculate this index, and find the following formula to be the simplest:

1. Multiply your weight in pounds by 700.
2. Square your height in inches (multiply your height in inches by itself).
3. Divide #1 by #2.
    For example:
    125 pounds x 700 = 87,500
    5'4"=64 inches x 64 = 4,096
    87,500 divided by 4,096 = 21.36

A BMI calculated in this matter should be 27 or lower to be in the healthy range. Women with a BMI above 27 are considered obese.

Now, calculate your BMI.

Your BMI is: _____ Date: _____

Your BMI is: _____ Date: _____

Hip-to-Waist Ratio

While the tendency for women to gain fat disproportionately in the buttocks, hips and thighs is unfortunate, it is actually more healthful than gaining fat in the torso, as most men do. The "apple" shape, which most overweight men possess, has virtually no waist and is more prone to obesity-related diseases than the "pear" shape. Part of the reason many women develop the "pear" shape is that we are programmed to accumulate less fat across the abdomen in order to facilitate pregnancy and childbirth. Instead of gaining it in the torso, it all goes to the lower body. This changes in midlife when women begin to gain weight in their upper bodies—with their child-bearing days behind them, there is no reason to spare the waist.

2. To further determine your health risk you need to look at your hip-to-waist ratio. Take your girth measurements at your navel and at the widest point of your hips, just over your buttocks. Divide your waist measurement by your hip measurement.

For example:

26-inch waist divided by 38-inch hips = .68

For most women, the hip-to-waist ratio should fall below .80 to be considered healthy.

Now, calculate your hip-to-waist ratio:

Your ratio is: _____Date: _____

Your ratio is: _____Date: _____

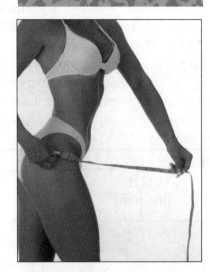

Keeping track of your health, weight and measurements is a great way to monitor your progress and stay motivated.

Lifestyle

3. To further determine health risk I ask my clients the following lifestyle questions:

1. Do you have high blood pressure, diabetes, osteoarthritis, high blood cholesterol or high blood triglycerides?
2. Does anyone in your family have any of these conditions or has anyone had heart disease?
3. Do you smoke cigarettes, overeat, drink more than one alcoholic drink per day or live with a high degree of stress?
4. Have you gained more than 15 pounds after age 25?

The Answer: If you answered yes to two or
more of the questions above, and if your BMI is more than 27 and

your hip-to-waist ratio is above .80, your health is in serious jeopardy because of your weight. A reduction in weight with the *Lower Body Solution* will begin to lower that risk immediately. Take these assessments again in two or three months and see how they've improved, along with your general health, energy and vitality.

What is Body Fat?

The scale measures your body weight. There is often a correlation between high body weight and high body fat. However, a very muscular woman may tip the scales at a heavy body weight but still have a very healthy body-fat ratio. Therefore, body fat is a better indication of a healthy weight than the scale.

There are several professional methods of determining body fat content that can be performed by a physician or health care provider. Three of the most popular are electrical impedance, skin calipers and underwater weighing. In lieu of professional testing, I have found the following self-test to be relatively accurate in determining body fat.

HIP GIRTH (INCHES)	PERCENT FAT	HEIGHT (INCHES)
32	10	72
	14	70
34	18	68
36	22	66
	26	64
38	30	62
40	34	60
	38	58
42	42	56

To use this chart you need two measurements: your height in inches and your hips, measured at the widest point, in inches. Then, take a ruler and set it at your hip girth measurement on the left side of the chart. Place the other end at your height measurement on the right column. Where the diagonal line of the ruler intersects the chart is your body fat percentage.

For women, 18-23 percent body fat is considered healthy. Over 32 percent is unhealthy and at risk of obesity-related disorders. Under 8 percent is too low and at high risk of diseases associated with malnutrition.

The Good News

The good news is that the exercise program in this book will begin immediately to diminish your risk of obesity-related disorders. Studies have shown that obese individuals who exercise regularly are less at risk of obesity-related diseases than obese people who do no exercise at all. Further, studies at the Mayo Clinic have shown that a reduction of just 10 to 20 percent in body weight that is kept off for at least three years will reduce the risk of disease by 25 to 75 percent!

I know you want to see results the first week. But, if you're trying to get stubborn fat off your body, you're going to have to be patient. Meanwhile, remind yourself of all the healthy things exercise will be doing for you as your body slowly moves into a "meltdown" zone where pounds will start to come off easier.

Heart disease is the number one killer of American women. It gets us after menopause when our protective estrogen supply has diminished. If you have a parent or sibling with heart disease, your risk goes up about 30 percent. Couch potatoes have about a 25 percent greater risk, as do overweight indi-

From *Sensible Fitness*, (second edition) by Jack Willmore, Ph.D. Copyright 1988 by Jack Willmore. Excerpted by permission of Human Kinetics, Champaign, IL. Out of print. Information on body fat measurements can be found in *Fitness and Health* (Fourth Edition) and *ACSM Fitness Book* (Third Edition). Both books are available in bookstores or by calling 1-800-747-4457, or by ordering on-line at http//www.humankinetics.com

viduals. The *Lower Body Solution* may dramatically lower your risk of cardiovascular disease.

This program may also lower your risk of breast cancer. One Norwegian study showed that women who exercised moderately for four hours per week were 37 percent less likely to develop the disease. Another report from the National Institutes of Health showed that non-exercisers were 20 to 50 percent more likely to suffer from high blood pressure, which affects 25 million American women. A Harvard study showed that people who reported high levels of physical activity had half the risk of colon cancer than their sedentary counterparts. Lastly, weight training has been shown to stimulate an increase in the density of our bones which helps prevent osteoporosis. Just being female puts you at risk: 80 percent of the 10 million Americans who have osteoporosis are women. After menopause, your risk increases dramatically. Weight training is one of the best ways to fight back.

The health benefits of this program are tenfold. Keep those benefits in mind as you work your way into the program. Weight loss will come; you've just got to give it time, especially when you're working on those stubborn pounds you've been lugging around for longer than you want to remember.

Goal Setting

When you set your weight loss goals, think small. One-half to one pound a week is reasonable. Tackle the first five pounds, then move your goal further up a notch. With each week of the exercise program you will have gained a mile toward better health, even if you've only shed a half-inch off your measurements!

I believe I have found a solution that can help any woman, whether she is 5 or 300 pounds overweight, to reduce her weight and achieve a better body than she believed possible. I wish the solution were as easy as turning to Chapter 13. However, you will need to read a few more pages to learn how to apply the *Lower Body Solution* to your personal weight and physique goals. But if you give it a try, I am confident you'll find the means to finally achieve the goals you've always dreamed of.

Welcome along on your journey to a new you.

Motivation

One thing is for certain: no one ever got in shape sitting around thinking about it. No one ever got in shape reading a book either. If the *Lower Body Solution* is going to work for you, you have to do it!

I have done everything possible to make this program user-friendly. There are photos of every exercise and precise instructions on how to perform them. There are three levels designed to accommodate your present level of fitness and special circumstances.

The *Lower Body Solution* workout, which actually begins in level three and lasts 16 weeks, is written to accommodate a busy lifestyle that may change from week to week. There are only three mandatory days in the health club each week. A fourth workout can be performed at home or the health club. Depending on how much you want to see a change, there are also two optional days.

On any given week you have a choice of working out from three to six days. Optimally, a program of this nature should vary between four, five and six days per week. Rather than structure the routine with those strict requirements, I give you the option. I don't expect you to work out six days a week for the entire 16 weeks. I expect things to come up where you may only make three or four of the workouts. I expect you may miss one entire week (which is okay, as long as you don't miss

three in a row, in which case you don't pass Go and must return to the beginning!). The home workouts can also be used for days when you may be out of town. The entire routine is set up around the life of a busy woman with more on her mind than getting to the gym.

Still, the getting to the gym part may be the most difficult aspect of this program.

Making a Commitment

Getting in shape means making a commitment. You need to give your workouts high priority. If going to the dry cleaners is more important than going to the health club, you're not going to succeed. How badly do you want to lose weight and get in shape? How badly do you want to wear a bikini? If you want a better body, and you want it badly enough, you'll put in the effort.

There are many "tricks" that can help motivate you. It's good to set a specific time each day for your workouts. Remember this is a "routine," so you should make it part of your daily routine.

Another good motivator is to buy a calendar and put it somewhere you will see it at your selected workout time. That may be the office, your kitchen or even the dash of your car. This calendar will keep track of your workout record. I use a big, bold marking pen and put a giant "W" on each day I work out. When I look back and see all the W's I've accumulated, I'm motivated to get even more W's! Also, if I miss three or four days in a row, seeing all that I accomplished before helps get me back in the gym rather than opting for the "oh well, I already missed four days, what's another four?" attitude.

You should keep your gym bag packed with clean workout clothes. Also, I keep a spare set of clothes and athletic shoes in the trunk of my car just in case I forget to grab my gym bag.

When you arrive at the gym it's also a good idea to wash your face with some cold water. This refreshes you and gives you a little jolt of energy to start your workout.

Set small goals at first. Sure, if you're just starting out, this is a seven-month routine (gasp!). But don't look at the total commitment, just take it two weeks at a time. In each two-week increment you will see positive changes in strength, endurance, sleeping habits, digestion, mood, energy, bodyweight and/or your physical dimensions. All these positive motivators will keep you incrementally on the program, and it will seem like only weeks when you look back on your calendar and glow at the months of W's you've collected!

Many people ask me about training at home. Yes, you could perform most of these workouts in a modified version at home. However, this program will be more successful if you join a health club. Why? Because you will have made a financial commitment with the purchase of a membership—and you will want to get your money's worth! Also, the variety of equipment at a health club will enable you to perform the more difficult routines and you'll see results faster than if you train at home.

Results are a powerful motivator. Set small goals for yourself (a half-inch or one or two pounds is a good starting point) and then keep

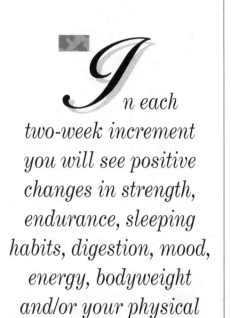

In each two-week increment you will see positive changes in strength, endurance, sleeping habits, digestion, mood, energy, bodyweight and/or your physical dimensions.

track of your progress. With every week, as you increase poundages and repetitions, note your improvements. Every time you see results, congratulate yourself and renew your commitment.

For me, training with a partner has always helped keep me on time and on the program. If you have a friend who will make the commitment with you, set up specific times to meet. When your workout hour nears you'll be less likely to beg off if you know someone is waiting for you.

I enjoy working out with other people. This is another reason I strongly recommend you join a health club. Even if you don't have a training partner, you'll meet other motivated people at the club and this interaction will make your workouts seem like more of a social activity than "work." As you start to see results, you'll be congratulated by others, and this again helps motivate you to stick with the program.

If this is the first time you've joined a health club, you may feel a bit intimidated. This is particularly true if you are out of shape. Try to remember that everyone in the club is there for the same reason as you, and many of them were out of shape at one time as well. If you make a commitment, you'll soon find that the health club is full of people who will be more than glad to share their own stories and advice. You'll make new friends, and you may find yourself a training partner as well.

Personal Trainers
Personal trainers work. They work because
a) you've made a financial commitment and
b) they are there to encourage you every step of the way.

Personal trainers make you feel important. A good trainer keeps you motivated, even on low-energy days. A great trainer carefully monitors your every move and constantly fine-tunes your program for maximum results.

The *Lower Body Solution* offers a certificate program for personal trainers to learn the nuances of this particular method. The certificate course is approved for continuing education credits from the American Council on Exercise, ACE. If you are looking for a trainer certified in this program or want to obtain certification for yourself, call 1-707-257-2348.

While I firmly believe personal trainers are an asset to anyone trying to get in shape, I have tried to write this book to take the place of a trainer. I myself like personal trainers, but not all of us can afford them, and not all of them are comfortable in accepting new programs like the *Lower Body Solution*.

Consider this book your own personal trainer. When you're doing your cardio sessions, reread some of the success stories. Peruse the exercise index and double-check that you're performing all the exercises correctly.

Each day follow the workout precisely, and write in your weights, times and some personal notes as you progress. Don't hesitate to make comments about portions of the workouts you enjoy, or don't enjoy. These notes will prove very useful when you finish week 16 of level three and start over again. Use this book as a workout journal and logbook. Simply looking back every few weeks will give you benchmarks of your own success on the program.

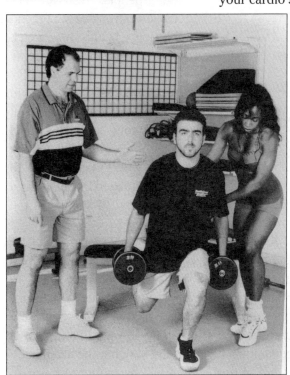

Coach Kim Goss,* with Lower Body Solution *personal trainers Dylan Leach and Tatiana Bryne, works on teaching lunge technique. Although this is a woman's program, Dylan and other male trainers are certified and very adept at teaching the method.

Choosing A Personal Trainer

If you want a personal trainer, and if a *Lower Body Solution* certified trainer is not available, there are still many great trainers who will help you with this program. Although the *Lower Body Solution* is presented in a precise format, a personal trainer will be invaluable in showing you how to properly perform each of the exercises. Unfortunately, finding the right personal trainer is like finding the right hairdresser. It takes time, and sometimes it's a process of trial and error. To help cut down on the error, here are four guidelines to aid you in your search.

1. **The best way to find a good trainer is through a personal referral.** If that option isn't available to you, contact the health clubs in your area. Some chains promote only their own trainers. A gym-employed or gym-certified trainer may be just what you want, but sometimes those trainers have less experi-

ence and motivation than the independents.

2. **Next, look at the trainer's longevity and experience.** If you're shelling out a hefty chunk of change for a service, there's no reason to wind up as a guinea pig for some beginner. You're paying to benefit from your trainer's experience, so make certain they have some! You may also want to ask for references.

3. **The person, and personality, count.** We have many men certified in the *Lower Body Solution*, so I don't believe it makes a difference whether you hire a man or a woman. You may feel more comfortable with one sex or the other. Your comfort is important because you will become "bonded" with your trainer in many ways. They are helping you along on an important journey that is closely tied to your self-esteem and confidence. Make certain the person you hire is someone you can share things with and one who makes you feel at ease.

4. **Arrange a one-week or one-month trial period.** Don't get hooked into a four-month contract. It is perfectly normal to ask for a trial period. Also, be certain to bring this book with you and make sure your trainer will work with you on your program, not theirs.

A Note of Thanks

I work out at HealthQuest Fitness and Martial Arts Center on Cabot Way in Napa, California. We have established a *Lower Body Solution* headquarters at the club, which was the first to offer my *Lower Body Solution* aerobics classes and the first to certify trainers in the method. I thank all the people who have put up with my photo sessions, my out-of-town visitors and my loud high-fives when someone new to the program has lost her first five pounds!

Particular thanks to Phil Andrews (for his endless supply of grapefruit fat-burner drinks) and to Jack and Karen Lair, for all their support, generosity and smiles. I'd also like to thank the entire staff for operating a health club that truly gives back to the community with a variety of programs and services for youth, the middle-aged and seniors; but mostly just for running a club where everyone is on a first-name basis.

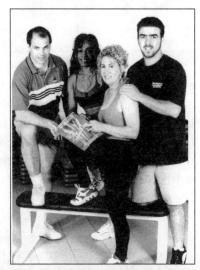

Special thanks to my Napa Valley-based crew Kim Goss, Tatiana Bryne and Dylan Leach for their support and contributions to the success of the Lower Body Solution.

Stubborn Fat
When you have 40-plus pounds to lose

This entire book is about losing fat. The following four chapters address the most stubborn kinds of fat: 40-plus pounds to lose, disproportionately large thighs which can only be slimmed with a six-day-per-week program, middle-age fat, and low-belly fat. You may be plagued by one, two or all three of these. If so, you will need to supplement the program with some special measures spelled out here that are designed to attack really stubborn fat.

40-Plus Pounds to Lose

One of the biggest hurdles to overcome if you have 40 or more pounds to lose is simply believing you can do it!

One of my clients, Marcia, wanted to lose 120 pounds to get back to her bodyweight of a decade ago. She is 5-foot-11 and "big boned." Her low belly is her worst spot, but she is lucky in that her fat is pretty well proportioned.

If I had a quarter for every time Marcia said to me, "My body is so used to this weight I don't think I can ever lose it," during those first two months, I'd be rich.

Marcia was a tough case because her diet had been very much out of control. She is a binge eater with an admitted addiction to particular foods, like ice cream and chocolate. The mere thought of "dieting" caused her to sit down and eat an entire large pizza, by herself, during her first week of workouts! Such behavior made it difficult to see any noticeable amount of weight loss in the first few weeks of the program.

If you have a lot of weight to lose, most likely your diet is also a bit out of control. We'll discuss strategies to get your diet under control later. But for now, don't even worry about trying to change your diet! Let's take things one step at a time. The first step is to start you on an exercise program. You can worry about changing your diet three months from now. Weight loss will occur with this exercise program alone, but it will be much slower than if you are able to follow the diet guidelines as well. The point is, weight reduction will occur!

If your weight is more a matter of sedentary lifestyle than diet, this program will have immediate and most gratifying results.

What to Expect

Many people believe if they have a lot of weight to lose that they will lose weight faster than a person with less weight to lose. Sorry, not true. Your rate of weight loss will be the same, and a weight loss of between one and two pounds a week is normal and healthy.

Depending on your diet, you may see weight reduction immediately on this program. However, many of you will begin the program on level one, which as explained later is a period to develop your baseline strength in order to perform the workouts that follow. Note that in the program there are certain modifications. These are built-in because you may be susceptible to knee injuries. If you have no pre-existing back or knee problems, you may be able to do the more difficult exercises. Experiment, but remember that any time an exercise requires you to work against the weight of your own body, you are working with a heavy load. Take special care with step-ups, squats, lunges and running. If you experience any pain or balance problems, definitely use the alternate exercises prescribed in the routine.

Take your weight and measurements at the start of the program, but be prepared to see only small increments in weight loss until you reach level two and three of the program. The first few weeks are designed to familiarize you with some of the equipment you're going to use. I know that you want to see immediate results, but that is not how this program is designed. It is set up for incremental but progressive and long-lasting results. This is a minimum six-month commitment, so be patient.

Your weight loss may also occur in spurts—you may lose four pounds one week and only one the next. This is because the program shifts its emphasis to keep your body from plateauing and to allow you to achieve steady, incremental weight loss over a period of several months.

If you use the alternate exercises remember that they are lower in intensity, and therefore produce weight loss at a slower pace. As you progress with the program two things will happen to help you speed up your weight loss. First, you will become better conditioned in order to put more intensity into your workouts. Second, the weight training will help increase your overall metabolism. As these two factors come into play, your weight loss will speed up.

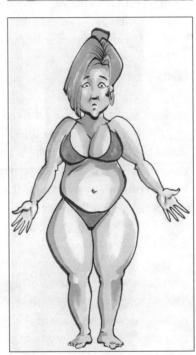

The more fat you've had, and the longer you've had it, the more stubborn it becomes. That's a fact. And that's why the Lower Body Solution offers you a six-day-a-week intensive fat-fighting arsenal to finally blast it away!

Metabolically, we are like snowflakes. No two people will react exactly the same, so I can only give you a general impression of how your weight loss may occur. What you must do is have faith that it will occur.

Marcia struggled on the program for nearly two months. Her eating habits improved subtly and her strength and conditioning improved drastically, but she only lost three pounds during the first five weeks. Fortunately, there were other positive benefits from the exercise which kept her on the program. She was sleeping better, had more energy, a better self-image because she was doing something positive about her weight and, lastly, she felt it was helping to stave off a lifelong battle she's waged with depression.

Fortunately, by week six Marcia began what I like to call the "melting" process. In the next three weeks she dropped more than ten pounds. The weight loss fueled her efforts to make some real changes in her diet and the quantities of food she ate, and over the next two months she managed to drop another eight pounds. Although still a long way from her ultimate goal, Marcia was well on her way.

Variety Is the Spice of Life

One of the many things that the Lower Body Solution does differently than conventional routines is to change the emphasis of the workouts every one or two weeks. As you progress with the program you will find a few of the routines work exceptionally well with your body. If this is the case, you may want to modify the program and perform that routine for an extra week—it won't change the total effects of the program and it will do you a world of good mentally.

Remember, however, you can't perform the same routine for more than three, possibly four weeks. At that point your body will adapt and you will not continue to see the weight loss you desire.

Emphasis on Aerobics

Additional aerobic exercise will contribute to faster weight loss. After the first three weeks you can begin to increase your aerobic workout times. Be careful not to overtrain. If you start to have trouble sleeping, low energy levels and a lack of desire to work out, chances are you're doing too much.

Your body will adapt to aerobics just as it adapts to weight training. When this happens, fat loss no longer occurs. Further, this can also result in overtraining, and one of the symptoms of overtraining can be an increase in body fat!

Exercise scientist Daniel Mercer is one of the world's foremost experts in aerobic training, having worked with many international-level track and field athletes. Instead of relying on just one standard aerobic training protocol, he has achieved success with a system called maximum aerobic power training (MAP). This system of hard work followed by easier work (or active rest intervals) is also known as interval training. We've adapted Mercer's interval workout principles and applied them to the *Lower Body Solution*.

However, if you desire maximum weight loss as fast as possible and choose to increase your aerobic times, you may need to interject a little "spice" into your aerobic sessions.

When you begin your level three workouts, or when you design your own workouts, you can replace every other cardio session with the following MAP training sessions. Perform these for a minimum of 20 minutes and strive to increase your times up to a maximum of 60 minutes.

When it comes to fat, MAP aerobic training is superior to traditional aerobic training. When performing hard work followed by easier work, you will momentarily elevate your heart rate beyond its "fat burning" zone into what is called the "cardiovascular zone." This is approximately 75-85% of your maximum heart rate. In other words, you'll be huffin' and puffin'. Here are three ways MAP can be applied during aerobic sessions.

Workout #1:
Treadmill, 30-45 minutes

Rather than power walking through this workout, try watching a clock in intervals. Begin with five minutes of comfortable walking as a warm-up.
- Perform 30 seconds of fast walking (almost running), followed by 60 seconds of slower walking (active rest) for approximately 15 minutes.
- Walk at a comfortable rate for five minutes before repeating this pattern.
- When you've completed your session, walk at a comfortable pace for five minutes to cool down.

Workout #2:
Stationary Bike, 30-45 minutes

The popular spinning classes today integrate Mercer's interval training principles. You can hold your own spinning class by cycling fast and slow in intervals. As with the treadmill workout, you will need either a timer on the bike, a wall clock with a second hand or a watch in order to keep track of the times.
- Perform 60 seconds of fast pedaling, followed by 120 seconds of slower pedaling, and repeat

this pattern for 5 intervals.

■ Pedal even slower for five minutes, before repeating.

■ Allow yourself a five minute warm-up and a five minute cool-down.

Workout #3:

Stairclimber, 30-45 minutes

■ Begin with a two minute warm-up.

■ Perform 30 seconds of fast stair climbing, followed by 60 seconds of slower stair climbing. Repeat this pattern five times, followed by two minutes of slow stair climbing.

■ For the second interval, perform 60 seconds of fast stair climbing followed by 120 seconds of slow stair climbing. Repeat this pattern three times.

■ Repeat these two 15-minute cycles for your allotted time and finish off with five minutes of slow stair climbing for your cool-down.

Much of the cardio equipment available today has a variety of intensity levels that will let you easily shift from the "hard" portions to the "active rest" phases of these routines. Some machines are also equipped with built-in "interval" programs that automatically do the same thing. Use the preprogrammed interval programs whenever possible.

Adding interval workouts into your cardio routine also keeps your workouts more mentally stimulating. One of the biggest drawbacks to aerobic training is that it can become boring. Interval training is one of the most effective ways to increase your interest in the program and burn maximum calories. Keep your cardio workouts interval based and you'll soon see those 40-plus pounds beginning to "melt" away!

Weighted Cardio

In addition to the MAP aerobic sessions you can also elevate your heartrate and reach your fat-burning zone quicker by incorporating weights into your treadmill sessions. Weighted work should not be added until you've reached at least level two of the program.

Use very light weights, one to three pounds at the most. Hold the dumbbells in your hands and "pump" your arms alternately with each step, like you see sprinters or race walkers doing.

To really bring your heart rate up, try "punching" straight out with the dumbbells as you walk. You'll feel your heart rate going up in half the time of your normal treadmill workouts. You probably won't be able to keep your arms going the entire session, so when your arms get tired, drop the weights to your sides for a minute or two to recover, then resume. If you begin to get too tired, feel dizzy or nauseous, carefully step off to the side of the treadmill and set the weights down.

These additional strategies will increase the total calories your burn during each workout and stimulate more dramatic weight loss. Incorporate them into your workouts every chance you get.

If you're truly applying yourself, you'll be able to tell by a quick check of your laundry basket. These workouts are designed to make you sweat and burn calories. If you're sweating enough to go through a clean T-shirt every workout, you're right on target!

You're Kidding!
Me? Work Out Six Days a Week to Slim My Thighs?

This may sound funny, but if your thigh measures larger than the diameter of your head, you are a good candidate for the *Lower Body Solution*. If it measures a lot larger than your head then you definitely need the *Lower Body Solution* to slim your thighs. So much for the funny part. The not-so-funny part is that the only way to slim disproportionately large thighs is to train them five or six days a week.

Got that, ladies? *Five or six days a week*.

I understand that for someone who hasn't been working out at all, that sounds impossible. I also understand that life gets in the way of five- and six-day-a-week workouts. That's why the workout program in this book has three mandatory workouts every week, and three optional ones. You must strive for the level three five- and six-day-a-week program, but when life gets too hectic, opt for a shorter version. The next week, try to get back on the five- and six-day-a-week program. That's how the program works.

However, I understand that some people will opt for the three-day-per-week version, every week. But if you really want to shrink big thighs, you can't afford that option.

For the Exercise-Resistant Mindset

As I said in Chapter 1, this book will work for women of all ages and all sizes. It will also work for those of you with exercise-resistant mindsets who think you can't train your legs five and six days per week—as long as you keep an open mind.

This chapter outlines five special workouts that can be done at home in fifteen minutes or less! Fifteen minutes is less than the amount of time you sit through commercials during the Monday night movie. If you live to be 75 you will have 2,534,400 opportunities to spend 15 minutes doing anything you want! All I ask is that you donate a few of those 15 minute slots to training your legs, and only for three weeks.

It's my hope you adapt the *Lower Body Solution* as an exercise lifestyle for the rest of your life; but for you hard-sell cases I only ask three weeks of your time on the level three program, using the following home workouts if you simply can't make it to the health club five or six days a week. Why three weeks? Because that's how long it will take to convince you that this program can work for you—even if you thought nothing could.

Before you begin, take your measurements. Measure your low belly at its widest points. Measure your hips and thighs at their widest point. To do this, stand facing straight on in front of a mirror.

When you measure again, be sure you are measuring from the same points.

Now, make a commitment to perform the *Lower Body Solution* five or six days a week for three weeks. That's all, just a three-week commitment. After three weeks, take your hip and thigh measurements again—I bet they're going to be less, by at least a half inch! If you achieve this much success, keep it up. You'll find the program truly works at fighting the female tendency to accumulate lower-body fat!

The Home Workouts

These programs are designed to be done at home. They are uniquely compliment the programs in Chapter 13 so that you will never use the same exercise, performed in precisely the same way, two days in a row. These routines are designed to be integrated into your *Lower Body Solution* level three program whenever you can't make it to the health club.

In other words: YOU HAVE NO EXCUSES!

These routines can be done in just a few minutes, anywhere. I often do them for "bonus" work in the evenings while watching the late news programs. Other times I might do them during the mid-afternoon on a weekend when I can't make it to the club.

Slow-Slow Training

To keep these routines effective, I've incorporated unique tempos. Tempo refers to the amount of time you spend completing each repetition and your rest between sets. A repetition is one complete exercise movement; a set is one group of exercise movements. Read the tempo times carefully and adhere to them. Many of these routines use a very slow tempo. This ultra-slow method of exercise puts a different tension on your muscles and keeps these routines from duplicating your regular *Lower Body Solution* exercise days.

This program uses compound movements in nearly every exercise. These are movements that work more than one muscle group, and burn maximum calories. They emphasize the lower body. I assume you will be following the program's three mandatory workouts in the health club; therefore,

you do not need many upper-body exercises in these routines.

The Lunge

One of the best fat-fighting exercise solutions is the lunge. Lunging exercises are compound, requiring the recruitment of every major lower-body muscle group. That means more muscle fibers are at work, and more calories are burned. More calories burned means you're melting off fat which, regardless of where it chooses to accumulate, is the root of the problem. Lunging routines, performed with fat-burning aerobic exercise on your three mandatory days, will have a dramatic effect on the lower-body fat that plagues so many women.

The toning action of the lunge works all the lower body muscles—the thighs, hamstrings and buttocks—to produce the long, lean limbs you see on ballerinas and figure skaters. Lunges are also easy to perform since you often do not need to add any additional resistance. Working against your body-weight alone usually puts you in the correct intensity zone to tone and sculpt, without adding excess size to your legs (which can occur when squatting or leg pressing heavy weights).

The lunge movement is also a functional movement. Some isolation exercises, such as the leg extension or the hamstring curl, work the muscles through a relatively small range of motion. The lunge, on the other hand, takes your lower body through a full range of motion that will translate to better running, jumping and sprinting strength.

Many people may be shocked by this high-frequency approach to training and initially think, "You can't train on consecutive days." Ask these same people why, and they'll complain about over-training, or worse, losing muscle size. Well, I'm all for losing size (muscle and otherwise) in the hips and thighs! As for overtraining, ask Olympic champion Jackie Joyner-Kersee if she suffers from training her legs every day! The fact is, those long-legged ballerinas, runners and skaters are all training six days a week and I don't see saddlebags on their thighs, or signs of overtraining!

It's important to vary the lunges in your routine, which is easy to do since there are so many variations to choose from. If you have pre-existing knee problems, avoid side-to-side lunges. Also, by leaning your torso forward slightly (not more than 10 degrees) you can remove much of the knee stress in forward lunges.

Even if you have no trouble balancing during lunges, it's a good idea to perform them near a wall or other support you can use for balance or a little assist. I prefer to do them next to a bench, sturdy chair or sofa, which I can also use for bench lunges and Gorsha lunges.

Here are five lower-body fat-fighter routines you can incorporate into your current workout program at home.

For complete explanations on how to perform each of these exercises, refer to the Exercise Index at the back of this book.

Lower Body Home Workouts

	Reps	Sets	Tempo (in seconds)
Workout One			
Lunge, Reverse	10 each leg	1	3 down, 2 up
Squat, Ballet	15	1	4 down, 2 up
Lunge, Reverse	10 each leg	1	3 down, 2 up
Squat, Ballet	15	1	5 down, 2 up
Pelvic Tilt	10	3	3 up, 1 down
Hamstring Stretch	12	2	5 seconds
Workout Two			
Combination Front and Side Lunge	*10 each leg	2	2 down, 2 up
Lunge Walk	60 seconds	1	2 down, 2 up
Lunge, Stationary	15 each leg	2	4 down, 2 up
Calf Stretch	12	2	5 seconds

*One lunge to the front followed by one lunge to the side constitutes one repetition.

	Reps	Sets	Tempo (in seconds)
Workout Three			
Plié, all 4 positions	8 each	1	6 down, 4 up
Squat, Ballet	10	1	3 down, 2 up
Ab Crunch	15	2	1 up, 2 down
Hip Flexor Stretch	12	2	5 seconds
Workout Four			
Lunge, Gorsha	10 each leg	1	3 down, 2 up
Lunge, Front	10 each leg	1	2 down, 2 up
Lunge, Gorsha	10 each leg	1	3 down, 2 up
Lunge, Side	10 each leg	1	2 down, 2 up
Petersen Step-Up	10 each leg	3	1 up, 2 down
Reverse Crunch	15	2	1 up, 2 down
Quadriceps Stretch	12	2	5 seconds
Workout Five			
Plié Position One	10	1	6 down, 4 up
Squat, Ballet	10	1	8 down, 6 up
Plié Position Two	10	1	6 down, 4 up
Squat, Ballet	10	1	8 down, 6 up
Plié Position Three	10	1	6 down, 4 up
Squat, Ballet	10	1	8 down, 6 up
Plié Position Four	10	1	6 down, 4 up
Pelvic Tilt	15	2	2 up, 2 down
Lower Back Stretch	11	2	30 seconds

Middle-Age Fat

As the baby boomers age, millions more people are wondering why their waistlines keep expanding. Is it an inevitable facet of age? Is it decreased activity? Is there anything that can be done about it?

Middle-age weight gain is a result of many factors. Overindulgence and reduced activity play key roles, but new research indicates that the problem is not entirely based in lifestyle. It appears weight gain is indeed an inevitable fact of aging; and for those who suffer from the condition, the only way to counter it is with diligent attention to diet and increased exercise. And while the formula sounds simple enough, the fact is that maintaining or regaining an ideal bodyweight in middle age is a complicated endeavor, filled with obstacles and trials.

One Woman's Battle

Cynthia Adams was on her high school cheerleading team in 1971. In the winter she snow skied and during the summer she swam and water-skied every chance she could. At 5-foot-4 her bodyweight hovered at 105 pounds, and she was used to relatives telling her she should put a few pounds on. She had a son when she was 27, and it took her less than four months to regain her pre-pregnancy weight and figure. When she was in her 30s friends would marvel at how she could indulge in a banana split and still weigh a svelte 110. At age 40 her weight was up to 120, but she was still one of the more slender mothers at her son's school. This fact didn't keep Cynthia from joining a health club and for the first time counting calories. The banana split was exchanged for a can of Slim Fast.

At age 44 Cynthia weighed 136, and all the weight had settled around her lower belly, hips and rear end.

"I'd never had to work at keeping my weight down, and suddenly it seemed like I was getting bigger by the minute," she recalls. "I was two sizes up in my jeans, and there was no way I'd put on a two-piece swimsuit. I was disgusted with myself, and it seemed like the more I tried to diet and exercise, the fatter I became!"

Cynthia was also experiencing the first signs of menopause. Her gynecologist told her that the reduced estrogen was changing the way her body stored fat, and thus the weight gain in her belly. Cynthia was also gaining weight in her upper body; it was just not as alarming to her as the belly bulge.

"Here I am at a time in my life when things

should be simpler. What happened to 'mellow-yellow?' Many things are easier—I don't stress over things. But when it comes to my weight it's getting tougher and tougher to stay the same," she says. "It seems unfair."

Cynthia is not alone in her dismay. While she was lucky to have enjoyed a slender figure most of her life, other women have had a constant battle of the bulge only to find the situation getting worse. A large part of the problem goes back to our genetic programming. Our bodies want to keep things status quo, and when estrogen levels drop with the beginning of menopause, the body counters this by storing more fat to maximize estrogen production. Just as menstrual cycles vary from one woman to the next, the amount of weight gain encountered at menopause varies as well.

What Happens During Middle Age

Whether you're a first-time fatty like Cynthia or someone who has battled the bulge her entire life, middle age (and older) is a whole new ballgame.

Age affects each of us differently. Part of what happens to us as we age is determined by our genes, and we can often look to our parents to foretell our futures. The way we age is also influenced by our lifestyles, and the effects of 40, 50 or 60 years of a particular lifestyle can often be very hard to turn around. Then there is the pervasive media that idolizes youth, making us feel that old age is best dealt with by airbrushing photos and by cosmetic surgeons.

The fact is, age changes how our bodies look and feel. We all want to look our best, but more importantly, we need to feel our best to enjoy not just longevity, but quality longevity. To that end we need to manage our weight and we need to preserve our muscle tone.

The first step to accomplishing these objectives is to arm ourselves with knowledge about what is happening to our bodies. Age affects us in different ways, but certain things can be expected. For example:

Illness— Heart disease is a major killer of men and post-menopausal women. Exercise—which is highly effective at burning fat—also helps fight off heart disease. Post-menopausal women are also at high risk for osteoporosis. Weight-bearing exercise has been shown to be effective at reducing this risk. Stationary bicycles and rowing machines are not weight-bearing exercise. Experts agree that the best weight-bearing exercise includes a combination of walking, running, stair-climbing, step aerobics, dancing and weight training.

Energy— Many older adults complain of a lack of energy. Illness, high fat-to-muscle ratios and excessive bodyweight can cause a general feeling of malaise; however, age in and of itself is not necessarily the culprit. If lack of energy is a concern, try a diet and exercise program to lower bodyweight, promote general good health and

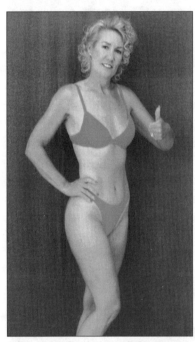

For me, losing weight at age 45 was a whole new ballgame. It was tougher than I ever expected, but I can also say I appreciated the results even more. There was a time early in my weight loss when I was ready to settle for the best I could look for a woman my age. Now, I see no reason why I can't continue to work toward the best shape of my life, for the rest of my life.

Lower Body Solution

decrease body fat, then watch your energy increase.

Skin Elasticity— Collagen is lost from our skin with age. Try this simple test. Take a pinch of skin from the top of your hand, let go and see how long it takes for your skin to return to its original shape. Now, perform the same test on someone less than 16 years old—the skin literally snaps back! There isn't much we can do to restore skin elasticity—short of cosmetic surgery. So, when you look in the mirror, remember that your skin tone—no matter how hard you workout and diet—is not going to be that of a 20-year-old.

Body Fat— A recent study at Lawrence Berkeley National Laboratory substantiated what Cynthia had already learned—increased fat is an inevitable part of aging. In a study of 4,769 male runners between the ages of 18 and 50, it was found that the average runner gained 3.3 pounds and about 3/4 inch around the waist each decade. The only way to prevent this weight gain is through diligent dieting or through increased levels of exercise. Another similar study is currently being conducted on women runners.

The Berkeley study is the first of its kind. Its findings contradict the exercise recommendations of the US Department of Agriculture's 1995 Dietary Guidelines of Americans that call for active individuals to maintain the same level of activity as they age. Although more study is necessary, those of us already in middle age may have to make our best assumption of the statistics and an educated guess as to how to take action rather than wait for the government to change its guidelines!

Menopause— Various theories abound about what happens to our fat storage during and after menopause. One interesting theory put forth by Debra Waterhouse in her book *Outsmarting The Middle-Age Fat Cell* is that as our estrogen stores are depleted as we go into menopause, our bodies fight back by increasing fat cell size in order to hold on to more fat. Fat is directly related to estrogen production. She equates this stage of life to being pregnant, when our bodies go into a fat-preservation mode for the sake of the fetus. If this is true, then as we go into the first stages of menopause (a condition that can affect us for ten years) we will need to increase efforts to keep fat off our body.

In addition, lowered estrogen changes the way in which our body stores fat. While pre-menopausal women store fat in the hips and thighs, lowered estrogen levels cause weight to accumulate in our low bellies. As we reach menopause weight is slowly shifted to our upper body. We also begin to store fat deeper and less in the subcutaneous region, just below the surface of the skin. In other words, we begin to store fat more like men. This means that upper-body exercise is going to be necessary to maintain muscle tone. It also means that we need to constantly fight the progressive weight gain. When we begin to gain weight in the same patterns as men, we also inherit

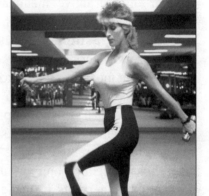

DeBarro Mayo, above, was my aerobics guru at Fit *magazine in the 1980s. Aerobics remain an important part of weight loss programs for women of any age.*

their higher risk of heart disease. Heart disease is the number one killer of women over the age of 55, and much of the risk is associated with our post-menopausal weight gain.

Many women opt to use Hormone Replacement Therapy (HRT) at the onset of menopause. HRT can cause weight gain or weight loss. Experience tells us that most women experience the same type of weight gain on HRT as they experienced on the Pill. Women on HRT often do not experience the changes in body fat distribution and composition described here. However, as my own gynecologist says, there are tradeoffs. HRT carries its own set of side effects, like weight gain, bleeding and water retention. Your decision to use HRT is one that must be made between you and your physician. Thankfully, there are also a number of alternative menopausal therapies available so we now have more choices than ever.

Body Composition— Muscle is lost as we age. This is why very old people are often cold— they lack the muscle tissue to keep them warm. As muscle tissue is lost, the ratio of fat to muscle is increased, causing a flabby appearance. Weight training can help maintain and restore muscle tissue and tone. Increased muscle mass has also been shown to reduce injury from falls and other mishaps for older adults. It should be an essential part of every middle-age workout.

Strength— Strength can reach its highest levels between the ages of 20 and 30, and begins to gradually decrease after that. The percentage of strength loss is greater in women than men, and is most pronounced in the lower body. Once again, more proof that weight training should be part of every woman's exercise routine in midlife.

Flexibility— Muscles shorten and stiffen with age. This lack of flexibility leaves older people more susceptible to injury during exercise and strenuous movements. Weight training should always be accompanied by a stretching routine, such as included here, to help elongate our muscles and keep us limber.

"Optional" Exercises for Older Women

If you're middle-aged or older you can follow the *Lower Body Solution* program. It is designed to work for you. As a middle-aged woman myself, I've made certain this program takes us into account at every opportunity. However, depending on your age and condition you may need to choose some of the less intense exercises listed as "options" in the workout. These easier exercises follow some of the more intense ones, and are listed in parenthesis in each of the workouts.

You also need to eat healthy. To make this task a little easier I rely on several supplements, the most important ones being those I purchase from U.S. Nutriceuticals (1-877-292-6614) under the Slim Again label. My favorites are the Weight Loss Shake and Diet Bar, both made from soy proteins and packed with a vitamin, mineral complex ideal for women in mid-life. Both of these can be used as meal replacements to help lower total calories and both contain special nutritional agents to enhance the body's natural fat-burning capabilities. Lastly, they taste really good.

The Most Important Thing

While supplements are valuable, the most important thing is exercise, exercise, exercise. You can reduce your chance of dying prematurely by almost half if you exercise every day or almost every day, according to sources at the Mayo Clinic. Regular physical activity cuts your risk of cardiovascular disease, some cancers, diabetes and osteoporosis—that's a fact. It also helps you control your weight, which not only lowers your risk of killer diseases, but of conditions such as arthritis which can be painful and exhausting. Regular exercise helps maintain your muscle strength, aerobic capacity and mobility so you can stay active and avoid injury as you age. And let's not forget that by boosting seratonin levels in the brain (your body's natural opiate) exercise can reduce stress, anxiety and depression.

Lose Belly Fat
Posture Tips to Make Belly Fat Disappear

*H*ere's a quick fix to instantly make yourself look better. Stand in front of a mirror in just your underwear, get comfortable, and really relax—you know, that kind of bored posture you might assume while waiting in a too-long grocery line behind a person with 22 rainchecks to redeem.

Now, turn to the side and look at the lines of your body. Are your shoulders slumped? Is your belly protruding? Is your head in a forward posture? These are the most common posture problems women suffer from. Slumped shoulders may be the result of attempting to divert attention from the front of our bodies: perhaps we try to cover large breasts or are overly conscious of small breasts. Or, it may be just years of poor posture. A protruding belly is probably the result of tilting the pelvis and "resting" on the spine, a posture exacerbated by wearing high heels. A forward head posture can result from too many hours spent at desk jobs and in front of computers.

Now, stand up tall as though you were lifting your head up through a crown. Bring your shoulders and head back, and rotate your pelvis so that your belt line is parallel to the floor.

You look noticeably better, right? Your lower belly even looks smaller. That's the beauty of good posture.

This chapter explores some of the ways you can permanently improve your posture for a better appearance and a stronger, pain-free back. To accomplish these goals you'll need to learn a bit more about the abdominals and the back. In so doing, you will not only learn how to achieve better posture and look as if you have a smaller belly, but actually lose some of that belly fat through better exercise mechanics.

The Battle of the Belly

The abdominals are of major concern to most women because of our genetic predisposition to gain fat in the lower portion of the belly. Further, during pregnancy the abdominal muscles become elongated and weakened and often require additional work to get them back in pre-pregnancy shape. And, all our muscles lose their elasticity with age. The sum total of age, pregnancy and a predisposition for storing fat in this area creates the perfect scenario for a paunched-out belly. What this means is that losing belly fat is a battle for us women, and we need to accept that it's not going to be easy.

Depending upon how you store fat, an overall reduction in body fat by itself often decreases the fat in your belly. In addition, exercise will tone and firm this area. Yet there is another very important key to resolving the embarrassment of a protruding belly: posture.

Many women have jobs that require a good deal of desk work. Computer work, in particular, creates bad posture habits. Most of us do not sit properly in front of computers, and further, we often poke our necks out like turtles to see the screen better. These conditions place unnatural stresses on the back and neck, and in time, muscle imbalances can occur that cause pain. If you work with computers, make certain your screen is directly at eye level and keep your neck in a neutral position; you should never have to look up and especially not down.

Another reason for slumped and forward-bent shoulders is that back and abdominal muscles work in pairs, so when one set of muscles develops an imbalance, the other set will as well. For example, if the pectorals are stronger than the upper back muscles, the shoulders will be pulled forward and the chest will look sunken. Women's high heels are another culprit in bad posture. Although heels may make legs appear longer and add pleasant curves to a torso, they do so by distorting natural posture. High heels force the entire torso forward, requiring small postural muscles to work extra hard to keep the body balanced.

We all remember falling sideways in heels when we were little girls, right? And if you think back, you'll probably remember finally mastering the art of walking gracefully in high heels somewhere in your late teens. What you did was "teach" your muscles a new sense of balance. Unfortunately, one of the repercussions of walking in high heels is that you train your muscles to function in an anatomically incorrect fashion. In turn, those small postural muscles develop imbalances, supporting structures become overstressed, and as an adult female you will most likely develop poor posture and suffer a bout or two of back or neck pain. Correcting this posture problem requires retraining those small muscles with very precise moves. It also requires time.

For most women a forward head posture and an excessive degree of pelvic tilt are the two biggest posture problems. These problems are commonly caused by poor flexibility in the hip muscles, and partly by a lack of development in the abdominal muscles and excessive tension in the lower back muscles. Are you now wondering why you should care so much about back muscles when we started this chapter talking about belly fat? Here's why: the consequence of having weak upper back muscles is poor posture—a posture in which the upper back is rounded, the shoulders droop forward and the chest is sunken. In order for you to maintain your center of gravity for this type of posture, the pelvis is rotated forward, causing a distended lower abdomen. This condition is often referred to as a kyphosis-lordosis posture.

In addition to causing the belly to stick out, poor posture also contributes to the formation of an unsightly hump in the upper back and

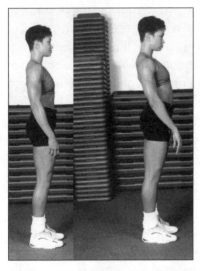

Lisa Lowe, above, demonstrates how good posture can improve one's appearance. Her erect posture at left causes her to look slimmer; while at right her swayback and forward head position looks awkward and less attractive.

neck region. Most of us associate this condition—the dowager's hump—with the lack of estrogen that comes with menopause which adversely affects the density of our bones. This is true, but poor posture can create a hump that is very similar in appearance to a dowager's. Further, a true Dowager's hump can be worsened by poor posture, and if left untreated can degenerate to the point where it cannot be corrected.

Correcting poor posture involves strengthening exercises both for the back and for the opposing muscles of the abdomen, as well as stretching. Although a medical diagnosis of your posture and precise corrective exercises should only be prescribed by a medical provider trained in this area, such as a chiropractor or a physical therapist, many of these medically-prescribed exercises are included in your *Lower Body Solution* workouts. Even if you are one of the fortunate few who do not suffer from poor posture, these exercises will help keep your postural muscles balanced, help you avoid back pain and injury, and also help you maintain lean, taut abdominal muscles for that "hardbody" look.

Posture is a habit. To improve your posture you'll need to learn better posture habits. That means reminding yourself throughout the day to sit and stand "tall." Also, remember to shift your pelvis so your beltline is parallel to the floor.

My posture problem is called a swayback. When I gained weight the condition worsened. When I saw a photo of myself I immediately realized I needed help. Thankfully, I found Clear Sky Products (1-888-CSP-2001), a company that offers something called a Spine Tuner that automatically reminds you of bad posture. The device comes in halter, bra-top and lumbar belt designs and is outfitted with a vibrating device that is activated whenever you slouch or hunch your back or shoulders. I use the shoulder halter to remind me to pull my shoulders back—I even wear it in the gym. Once I pull my shoulders back, I'm reminded to tilt my pelvis so my beltline is parallel to the floor, correcting my swayback. These devices are fully adjustable and provide you with instant feedback. I recommend them heartily to anyone who wants to relearn better posture.

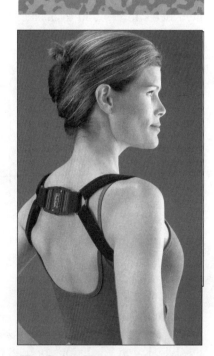

The Spine Tuner is a device that vibrates to remind you to stand straight and keep your shoulders back.

Practical Posture Tips

Studies show that up to 85 percent of all Americans will have back pain at some time in their lives. Some theorists attribute this to the fact that we stand on two legs—they claim that our backs would be much stronger if we walked on all fours, as dogs do. However, it is also a fact that four-legged animals have an inherent structural weakness in the middle of their spines. Regardless of whether you believe the human spine was designed to be horizontal or vertical, walking on all fours is simply not a viable solution to the problem! Better posture and exercise techniques are.

Training the postural muscles of the back is always difficult because, well, they are in the back. It is much easier to train muscles in the front of the body where you can see and enjoy them working.

Over-attention to the muscles in the front of the body is one of the reasons so many women suffer from poor posture in the first place. Overworking the upper abdominals, chest and shoulders in conventional routines forces the shoulders to round and the chest to sink so that the body sort of "caves in" on itself.

One immediate improvement you can make is to limit the amount of time you spend in high-heeled shoes. Wearing high heels forces you to make considerable corrections to your posture with exaggerated back curves and unnatural bending in the knees. Heels also force most of your bodyweight to shift towards the front of the foot, a condition that can disfigure toes and may cause painful bunions and bone spurs. The solution is to buy shoes with low or no heels. Wearing comfortable shoes also encourages you to move around during the day, increasing the total calories you burn and reinforcing a mindset that encourages a healthy, active lifestyle. Karen Voight, one of the fittest women in the world, says she wears sneakers every day just so she never has an excuse not to jog up a flight of stairs!

Another bad posture habit many women practice is to "collapse" when standing at rest. The perfect time to observe this is while standing in the supermarket checkout line. While waiting, many people will lock their knees, extend their pelvis and allow their upper bodyweight to "rest" on their spine. This posture will cause the spine to literally compress after many years, creating degeneration of the supporting structures of the spine. Instead, when standing relaxed, make it a habit to use your back and abdominal muscles to hold your torso upright. It may not be quite as comfortable at first, but this posture habit will make you look better and improve the condition of your spine for a lifetime.

If you have a desk job, you can easily make some improvements in your posture while at work. Make certain your chair allows you to sit straight, with your feet flat on the floor. If you work with a computer screen, make sure it is positioned at eye level—you should not have to look up or down to see your screen.

Posture is a habit. Improving your posture requires you to develop a new, good habit. This means you will have to continually remind yourself to hold your body in the correct position. At first, practice correct posture in the mirror. Turn to the front and side to make certain that you have your body aligned properly. Your head should be over your shoulders; your shoulders and hips should be in line, and your bodyweight should be distributed evenly to rest in the middle of your feet.

It's a good idea to have posture checks throughout the day. To make this easy, practice the "nine-twelve-three-six routine." Every three hours, check that you are holding your body in good posture—wherever you are, at your desk, in your car, at the health club, and at the dinner table. Eventually, naturally good posture will return to you as you develop your new habit.

Lower Body Solution Abdominal Training

While correct posture can give the appearance of a flatter belly, nothing replaces good abdominal

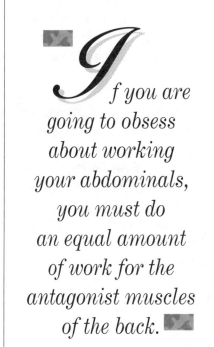

If you are going to obsess about working your abdominals, you must do an equal amount of work for the antagonist muscles of the back.

training techniques and a sound program of exercise for maximum caloric expenditure to get your mid-torso in shape.

Abdominal exercise is not a fabulous calorie burner, unlike most lower body exercise. As a matter of fact, it would take tens of thousands of sit-ups to burn off the calories contained in just one teeny little chocolate truffle. However, just as high-frequency lower body training contributes to a decrease in body size, proper abdominal training will lead to a tightening of the abdominal region through improved muscle tone. When teamed with a fat-burning program such as the *Lower Body Solution* and with improved posture, the result will be a tight, flat and toned waistline.

One of the most important principles of abdominal training is to have balance—this includes attention to both the lower and upper areas. And although too much emphasis on the obliques can contribute to a blocky waist, some attention is mandated. Those who rely only on crunch movements will not develop the lower abdominal strength to counteract the pull of the hip flexors. What results is the upper region becoming short and chronically tense, and the lower region becoming long and weak. This imbalance encourages an unflattering posture characterized by a forward tilt of the pelvis and excessive curvature in the lower back.

Principles of Abdominal Training

Conventional sit-ups have probably done more harm to abdominals than chocolate! The abdominals are a highly evolved network of muscular fibers that work together to provide stability and movement of the torso. It's not that the sit-up is altogether bad, but relying solely on this exercise is counterproductive because it will create muscle imbalances. To be sure you are using proper technique, follow these guidelines:

1. **Be aware of head posture.** One of the functions of the abs is to pull your shoulders toward your knees—not to pull your chin or head forward. I do not advocate placing your hands behind your head to pull the head toward your knees. This uses momentum instead of control

and strength, may cause neck pain, and forces your upper back and neck muscles to contract to stabilize your shoulders. When you perform abdominal work, slightly retract (pull back) your chin and keep your chin away from your chest. Instead of placing your hands behind your head, place them at your sides when possible.

2. **Avoid neck fatigue with proper tongue placement.** Perform ab work with your tongue resting on the roof of your mouth, just behind the front teeth. Paul Chek, a popular lecturer who gives extensive workshops on abdominal and back training, deserves credit for discovering this important concept. According to Chek, the roof of your mouth just behind the front teeth is the anatomical resting place of the tongue. When the tongue is in this position, the proper muscles of the neck handle the stress and optimal training is possible. Chek says this technique may even prevent tension headaches!

3. **Use a full range of motion.** Full range of motion on many abdominal exercises means resting the entire weight of the head on the floor between each repetition, which will allow the neck muscles to relax and thereby help prevent neck strain.

4. **Avoid performing only bent-leg abdominal exercises.** Some exercise instructors believe that by bending the knees you will effectively isolate the upper abs. This is not true, and it has been shown through electromiocardiogram (EMG) studies that for the first 30 degrees of movement there is no safety advantage between sit-ups with either straight or bent legs. Also, performing only bent-leg exercises will tend to tighten and shorten the hip flexor muscles. This leads to muscle imbalances that may decrease flexibility, especially in the groin area, and adversely affects the proper biomechanics of walking, running and jumping.

5. **Do not anchor the feet.** Using sit-up boards with supports for your feet, or holding your partner's feet, will encourage the hip flexor muscles to become involved earlier than wanted during the exercise. This effect will significantly increase stress on the lower back.

6. **Always inhale at the start of an abdominal exercise and exhale at the top of the movement.** Exhaling while performing the crunch (or curl-up movement) reduces tension on the oblique muscles. However, holding your breath too long causes a dramatic increase in blood pressure.

7. **Perform slow, precise movements unless directed otherwise.** The abdominal exercises presented in the *Lower Body Solution* tend to be safer and work the muscles harder when performed slowly and without sudden or bouncing movements.

8. **Rotation for oblique exercises should start at the beginning of any abdominal exercise.** Remember Rocky doing sit-ups in the gym and violently twisting at the top? This makes for exciting cinema, but the fact is that waiting until the movement is complete before twisting reduces the effectiveness of the exercise. Simultaneously lifting and rotating is ideal.

9. **Proper use of abdominal machines is essential.** Seated trunk twisting machines can create excessive stress on the discs and spinal ligaments, and the standing machines can place excessive stress on the knees and lower back. Seated crunch machines can also create problems. Using too much weight can strain muscles. Having a seat too high increases lumbar curvature, and having a seat too low increases the relative weight being lifted.

10. **Perform lower abdominal exercises first.** When I speak of lower abs, I'm referring to the external obliques. These are attached to the pelvis; and when they contract they rotate the pelvis backward—in contrast to the hip flexors, which rotate the pelvis forward. Because the upper abdominal muscles provide stability for many lower abdominal exercises, for optimal performance it's important not to fatigue the upper abdominals first.

Achieving a tight midsection with enviable and dramatic definition will require both a decrease in body fat and an increase in abdominal conditioning. You simply can't achieve great abs with one and not the other. Therefore, as you begin the *Lower Body Solution* program, be mindful of the fact that until you effectively reduce body fat, sleek abdominals are not going to appear.

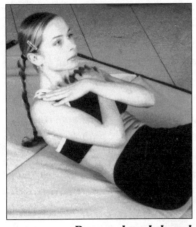

Proper head, hand and tongue position is necessary in order to get maximum results from performing abdominal crunches and sit-ups.

Aerobic Meltdown

*W*hat would a woman's exercise book be that didn't address aerobics? Face it, aerobics are a woman's exercise. We like aerobics. We're good at aerobic exercise. Aerobic dance is fun.

While there are normally vast differences in strength levels between men and women, when it comes to long-distance endurance, we women are as tough as our male counterparts, maybe even tougher. And as we grow older, we get better. Did you know that female distance runners don't hit their peak until their mid 30s, and some of the top women runners are in their 40s?

Aerobics, or cardiovascular training ("cardio" for short), requires the use of oxygen, whereas anaerobic training (like weightlifting) does not. Another difference, and one that is especially important if you're trying to lose weight, is that the aerobic system primarily uses fat as its energy source, whereas anaerobic exercise favors carbohydrates. Because women can burn fat more efficiently than men can during aerobic exercise, this form of exercise is particularly valuable for women as a means of weight control.

The type of energy system (aerobic vs. anaerobic) used when you exercise is determined by the duration and the intensity (degree of difficulty) of the activity performed. The aerobic system is the primary energy source in activities that are low in intensity but long in duration. The anaerobic system is the primary energy source in activities that are high in intensity but short in duration. As a general rule, any activity that is completed within two minutes is considered anaerobic, and any activity that continues for more than two minutes is considered aerobic. Thus, lifting weights is an anaerobic activity and jogging a mile is an aerobic activity.

The *Lower Body Solution* program assumes you want to lose fat and bodyweight and therefore aerobic workouts are planned throughout. If you need to lose 20 percent or more of your total bodyweight, you may want to increase the cardio times prescribed. If you don't want to lose bodyweight, you may want to decrease the times.

The *Lower Body Solution* is a total program and can be performed as your sole form of exercise. If you live a normally active life, continue all your activities. The bad news is, if you're one of those women who presently live for your morning step classes *and* evening boxercise sessions three or four times a week, you may have to give those up. Performing this routine in addition to large amounts of supplementary cardio will increase your risk of overtraining and can diminish your results. The good news is that if you've been a "cardio-machine" for quite some time and are not seeing the results you want to see, this program is most definitely the answer.

Which Type of Cardio Is Best?

Although exercise physiologists are still debating this issue, the bottom line is that all types of aerobic exercise can help you achieve your fitness goals. If you like to walk, walk. If you like aerobic dance, dance. If you like to swim, swim. For the record, the treadmill usually rates highest at the gym because it easily provides various levels to work at and causes minimal stress to the joints. For people with bad knees or excessive weight, and who require even less impact on the ankles and knees, the recumbent stationary bike is preferred.

Stair climbing machines are great for working the lower body; however, you must avoid the tendency to "cheat" on these machines. Use the handrails for balance only. Do not lean on them to support your bodyweight because this drastically reduces the effectiveness of the exercise. To get the most out of your stairclimbing, stand upright with your arms at your side. My favorite stair climbing machine is called the Climbing System by StairMaster. Instead of rails at your sides it has two "handles" at head-height to use for balance. I find "cheating" much more difficult on these machines. They are also preprogrammed with an excellent interval program (Program Seven) that I use several times a week.

Almost all machines are equipped with these preset programs. Interval training, where short bursts of hard work are followed by periods of lesser intensity, is the most effective at burning fat. When these programs are available, use them.

The *Lower Body Solution* routines usually specify which type of cardio you should do. However, you can make substitutions depending on the equipment available and your present level of conditioning.

Just as weight training exercises must vary to keep producing results in your workout, your aerobic training needs to vary as well. In fact, one of the primary reasons many women don't achieve the results they want from aerobics is that they remain on the same exercise for too long and create a state of overtraining that causes them to hold on to their fat. Therefore, you'll notice in the *Lower Body Solution* program that you will frequently either change the activity or alter the duration or intensity. If you make substitutions, be certain to vary intensities.

As you increase your conditioning level on this program you will also decrease the amount of time it takes your body to reach its optimal fat-burning zone. Therefore, even though the amount of time you spend is relatively constant, as you progress in the program your efficiency will increase. At first it may take you 30 minutes to hit your fat-burning zone. In four weeks' time it may only take you 15 minutes.

An amazing example of this principle was demonstrated by long distance runner Alberto Salazar. In his prime, his body began burning fat for fuel less than 45 seconds into his run!

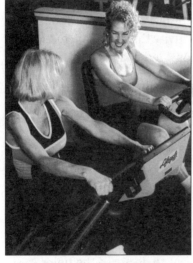

For maximum weight loss, you may want to add an additional 10-20 minutes of cardio time, several times a week, to your exercise routines in level three. The recumbent cycle, which Patty Atkinson and I are using in this photo, is excellent for anyone with weak knees or with 40 pounds or more to lose.

Intensity Is Key

The media frequently cites studies that indicate any amount of exercise has a benefit. Of course, every magazine editor loves a cover teaser that says "5 Minutes of Walking Is All You Need!" Five minutes of walking may be beneficial for individuals who have never exercised on a regimented program. However, once you've established a base level of conditioning, the intensity level of your workout—whether weight training or aerobics—dictates the results you will obtain. While "no pain, no gain" may be a bit hardcore, "no effort, no effect" is quite accurate.

Intensity is key to using aerobic exercise for fat loss. At low intensity you are just using up a little energy. At 60 to 80 percent intensity you are burning fat calories, and those are the calories you want to burn. At higher intensities you go into what's called the "cardio zone" and your body is using other energy sources as well as producing lactic acid. If performed excessively, high-intensity exercise compromises your optimal fat-burning ability. Therefore, finding your fat-burning zone is very important if you're using aerobic exercise to lose weight.

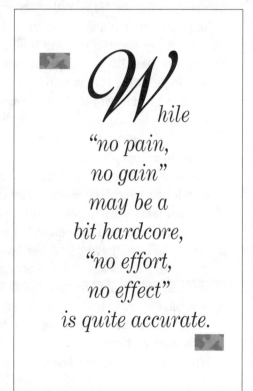

While "no pain, no gain" may be a bit hardcore, "no effort, no effect" is quite accurate.

Know Your Heart Rate

Many treadmills and stationary bikes are equipped with heart rate monitors and charts that tell you when you're in the optimal fat-burning zone. It usually takes a few minutes to reach your target heart rate that puts you in your most efficient fat-burning zone. The amount of time it takes depends on your present conditioning, body composition and the intensity of the exercise you are performing. On average, it will take about 20 minutes to reach this most effective fat-burning zone.

Most people follow the general guidelines promoted by organizations that certify personal trainers, such as the American Council on Exercise or the American College of Sports Medicine, for determining their heart rate and fat-burning zone. You'll often see aerobic classes with wall charts that list these guidelines. Most cardio machines have abbreviated charts showing your fat-burning zone and safe heart rate.

Maximum heart rate (MHR) is the determining factor in gauging the intensity of aerobic activity. Professional testing, preferably by an exercise physiologist or physician, is considered the safest and most reliable way to determine your MHR, but there are also formulas that have been used to estimate this number. One popular formula simply has you subtract your age from 220. For example, a 20-year-old would have a MHR of 200 (220 - 20 = 200).

During aerobic exercise, an intensity level of 60 to 75 percent of your MHR is considered best for fat burning, with beginners usually advised to stay at the lower end of the range. You can monitor your heart rate with frequent pulse checks by using a heart rate monitoring device. Because exercising to music often makes an activity seem easier than it is, it's recommended that you frequently check your pulse rate to make certain you're exercising at the appropriate intensity level.

In addition to built-in machine monitors, there are also wrist, finger and chest monitors you can purchase that will tell you your heart rate during exercise. Polar heart rate monitors (1-800-227-1314) are excellent products that I recommend. They are a good investment because the individual monitors are more precise than the built-in ones.

A simple way to gauge your aerobic intensity level is the Talk Test. You should be able to speak in a normal, conversational voice (without gasping for air) during cardio exercise. The exception to this rule is during the intense portions of interval cardio training.

Another gauge of aerobic intensity is called Perceived Rate of Exertion (PRE). Imagine that 10 is really putting everything into your exercise. Using that as a measure, your aerobic zone is 6-8, or 60 to 80 percent of your MHR.

Of course, you may want to get your cardio exercise performing an outdoor activity, such as skating, jogging or bicycling. I love to bicycle around the Napa Valley—the views are wonderful and the rolling hills give me a great workout. I also like the fact that I can't slouch on my aerobic training times: if I pedal a half-hour north, there's no way back except to pedal another half-hour home. Interestingly, while I think nothing of 50-mile bicycle rides, I dread stationary bicycle workouts and wear out within ten minutes on level one. Go figure.

In general, a few other rules about aerobic exercise should be adhered to in this program:

1. When combining aerobics with a weight training routine, perform your longest aerobic sessions after the weight training. This helps prevent large muscle gains from weight training more effectively than if you perform the cardio beforehand.
2. Once you've achieved a higher level of aerobic fitness, you can trim your cardio sessions to about one-third the time commitment and still maintain that fitness level for several months.
3. Aerobic exercise should not exceed one hour in a single workout session—its effectiveness as a fat-burner is decreased substantially after an hour.

Which brings us to our last cardio topic.

Is There Such A Thing As Too Much?

Yes! Jack LaLanne once said that "everything should be in moderation." That was great advice 30 years ago, and it's still great advice today. Too much exercise—whether aerobic or anaerobic—can result in overtraining, which can lead to chronic fatigue and illness.

When you achieve a reasonable bodyweight and fat-to-muscle ratio, you can ease up on the amount of cardio exercise you perform. Again, you will need only one-third the time commitment it took to obtain your level of aerobic fitness in order to maintain it.

The *Lower Body Solution* cardio program is designed so that you lose weight, but don't overdo it. If you follow the program precisely, you should achieve maximum weight loss. However, if you add aerobic sessions to those prescribed, you need to be careful that you don't overtrain. Signs of too much cardio exercise include:

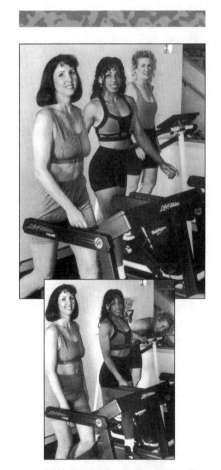

I like to mix up my cardio sessions between the treadmill, stationary bike and stairclimber. When using the stairclimber, avoid using the rails to support your weight— and never lean over the machine, as I so aptly demonstrate above.

- Tired all the time
- General malaise
- Difficulty sleeping
- Weight plateaus
- Weight gain

If you experience any of these symptoms you should cut back on your cardio. I've known many women, and I've seen hundreds more in health clubs, who continue to do hours of cardio when their bodies look emaciated. An addiction to aerobic exercise is almost as unhealthy as getting no exercise at all! Remember that aerobic exercise should form a part of your exercise program but should not overwhelm it.

Weight loss of one or two pounds a week is the most you should aim for. Remember, if it took a long time to put on those extra pounds, it will take time to take them off safely and permanently. Be patient.

CHAPTER ELEVEN

First-Time Lifters

If this is the first time you've ever worked out with weights, then there are several "basics" we need to cover before you begin the program.

First of all, lifting weights requires effort. But don't be afraid of building muscle size. This program assumes that you want muscle tone and the subsequent curves, not mass. Absolutely everything has been designed in this program so that you do not put on muscle size. Later I'll explain how and why this program can use weight training for weight loss, not size. For the moment, just trust me that you can exert effort, even experience a little of what bodybuilders call a "pump," but not grow large muscle.

How Much Do I Lift?

The first question most people want answered when they begin weight training is "How much do I lift?" Unfortunately, that's one question that doesn't have a simple answer.

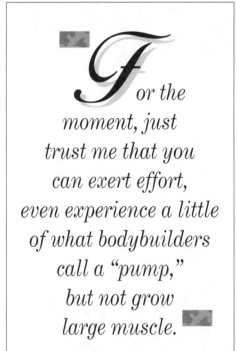

For the moment, just trust me that you can exert effort, even experience a little of what bodybuilders call a "pump," but not grow large muscle.

Muscular strength is a funny thing. At first it appears to defy logic; after a time, you'll find some rules that help you understand it.

First of all, there's a "beginner's luck" syndrome to weight lifting. You may find that your first attempts allow you to lift far more weight than later attempts. That may be a little disappointing during your first few sessions, but after a few weeks you'll develop real strength gains and see a progressive increase in the weight you can lift.

I attribute the beginner's luck syndrome to the fact that muscles have "memory." When you first attempt to lift a weight, your muscles don't know what's in store and they jump to attention. That's why first-timers usually start out lifting quite well. The next time you attempt that same weight stack your muscles know what they're in for, and they back off. Just as in riding a horse, you have to tell your muscles who is in charge. That's where the effort comes in.

When I lift weights I begin each exercise by

pausing for a moment to rehearse the movement in my mind. Sometimes, I "pace for power." I look down at the floor, consciously eliminating the health club movement and noise from my mind, and pace back and forth "collecting" my mental focus. Then I lift. If the first two repetitions feel too light, or too heavy, I make an adjustment.

It's important to think about the specific muscles each exercise targets. I can't tell you how many people have told me that their arms are doing all the work when they bench press when, in fact, it's the chest and shoulders that are being emphasized. In the Exercise Index at the back of this book each exercise lists the specific muscles it works. Before you perform the exercise, stop and think about that muscle. If it works the chest, back or legs, remind yourself that these are the biggest and strongest muscle groups in your body and capable of strength far beyond what you probably believe you can achieve.

Limit Strength

In the world of weights there is a term called "limit" strength. This refers to the maximum amount of exertion your muscle could possibly achieve. To prevent us from tearing our muscles from their attachments, we mentally stop ourselves from using our limit strength.

Here's a story that illustrates this point well: While changing a tire, a woman watched in horror as the carjack failed and the weight of the entire car crashed down upon her child, who had crawled under the vehicle when she wasn't looking. Without thinking, she lifted the car to save her child. I don't know the authenticity of the story, but it has been told so many times it must have some truth. The explanation for such strength, which I truly believe we are capable of, lies in part in the fact that the woman was experiencing "beginner's luck." Moreover, her emotional reaction overpowered her body's instincts to temper muscular exertion and allowed her to access her limit strength.

I explain this because so many women, particularly those who have not weight trained before, believe they can lift only minuscule weights. While a woman's upper body strength is much lower than a man's, her lower body strength is actually quite comparable. However, with training women can become quite strong overall.

Finding Your Ideal Lifting Weight

When it comes to how much weight you should lift, I have no answer because every individual is different, every lift is different, and every machine is different. Just because you leg press 90 pounds on one machine doesn't mean that you can go to another health club's machine and do the same weight. It also doesn't mean that

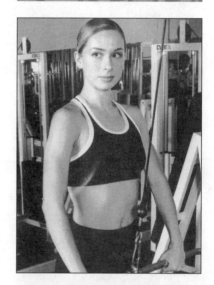

"Limit" strength refers to the maximum exertion your muscles are capable of. Most women are not accustomed to using anywhere near their limit strength. As a matter of fact, most women think of lifting only miniscule weights. As you begin weight training you will most likely be surprised at how strong you are, and how quickly you become noticeably stronger.

you can squat 90 pounds. Every time you switch exercises or machines, you must start from ground zero to determine your individual lifting weight.

When you first begin an exercise, choose a low poundage or machine setting. Perform one or two repetitions, and see if the weight provides some resistance or effort to lift. If not, increase to a higher poundage. The ideal weight for you to lift should require some effort for you to perform the first six to eight repetitions, and additional effort to complete repetitions nine and ten. If you are performing three sets, the weight you use should require considerable effort to complete the third set.

Weight training is called "progressive resistance exercise" because the process is progressive. Although you'll reach a point where you level off, for the first few months you'll be changing weights with every workout as you find your optimal strength levels. The good news is that once you've done this a few times, it usually takes a single warm-up set to find the weight you should be lifting that day.

Weight Training for Weight Loss

This book is about using weight training for weight loss. Studies have proven that reduced-calorie diets are the fastest way to lose weight. Therefore, a reduction in calories will be necessary to see fast and dramatic weight loss. However, weight training is going to contribute to your weight loss in many significant ways.

Weight training takes a little longer than diet to accomplish weight loss, but the effects are more permanent. At the beginning of your program, weight training will help you lose weight because it increases the number of calories you burn in a given day even while your body is resting. As you increase your base level of fitness, weight training will begin to build a degree of muscle that will increase your metabolism. When you increase your metabolism, you burn more calories even while at rest. This will help you keep the weight off and avoid the Yo-Yo diet syndrome of weight loss and weight gain.

While studies show that dieting is the single quickest method to lose weight, follow-up studies show that when dieting is used as the only form of weight control, the rate of weight regained is nearly 100 percent in almost 90 percent of dieters! In contrast, when exercise is used as a method to lose weight, and that exercise program is continued after weight loss occurs, the majority of individuals manage to keep the weight off because of the metabolic changes exercise creates!

There are other important reasons why women should weight train. Weight training can strengthen muscles and bones, and studies have shown that programs such as these can lower the risk of developing osteoporosis, the brittle-bone disease. Studies have also shown that weight training programs boost self-esteem and aid sleep. I can tell you from firsthand experience that weight training will make you stronger and more confident in performing physical tasks. Further, when performed properly, weight training will improve your posture and prevent a great deal of back, neck and knee pain.

Of course, weight training will also add muscle tone to your body. Tone, mind you, not big muscle. This will help firm up flabby skin. The appearance of cellulite can be reduced. Pleasant curves can be built. Basically, a woman's feminine shape will be positively enhanced in every way.

Why You Won't Build Muscle
You hear just about everything in the fitness industry. We've already discussed the misguided theory that weight training will cause large muscle growth in women. There is also a contingent who believe that women are incapable of building large muscle without the use of drugs, so not to worry.

Wrong.

Anyone who says a woman can't build big muscle naturally hasn't been around the sport of women's bodybuilding as long as I have. Depending on a woman's body type and hormone levels, she can build a lot of muscle, or a little. But it's absolute malarkey that estrogen prohibits women from building large muscle. Sure, some of the most grotesque women bodybuilders have used steroids to achieve their massive physiques, but don't kid yourself thinking that a woman can't build muscle naturally through weight training.

The *Lower Body Solution* assumes that you do not desire large muscles. Therefore, the program has several safeguards built in to ensure that you DO NOT build big muscles. I'd like to quickly review these safeguards in the hope that I can convince you, beyond any doubt, that this program will not build muscle size. This is a very important point to understand, because I will be asking you to lift weights with some real effort, sometimes teeth-clenching effort that may even have you groaning like a powerlifter! The effort is necessary, but you can rest assured that it will not result in overly developed muscles.

Here is a checklist of safeguards built into this program to ensure lean body mass development without large size:

■ You will exercise with weights that use about 65 to 75 percent of your total strength threshold. Large muscle growth is induced by heavy weightlifting—lighter loads do not pack on the bulk.

■ Aerobic exercise is performed at the end of your weight training program. Aerobics compromise your body's ability to build muscle when performed at the end of a routine.

■ Compound movements that require several muscle groups to perform are used instead of isolation movements designed to develop the smaller, showy muscles that bodybuilders so proudly display.

■ You will exercise using short rest intervals to increase the levels of growth hormone, an important naturally occurring hormone that helps you burn fat.

■ You will exercise the same muscle groups frequently. By exercising the same muscle four, five or even six days a week, the muscle will not respond with a noticeable increase in size, but you can enjoy the resultant calorie burn.

■ You will alternate exercises so that body parts are not exercised consecutively in the same routine—this prevents excessive lactic acid buildup and the subsequent soreness that can occur when training on a high-frequency program.

Routines Just for Women

Think about your overall physique goals. Once you've completed level three of the program you'll be ready to fine-tune your weight

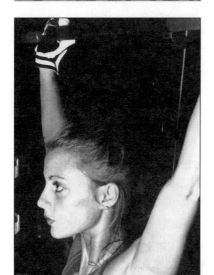

In the past, weight training has been thought of as a means to build muscle and gain size. The Lower Body Solution program uses weight training to lose fat and tone muscle.

training program. Do you want a rippled abdominal section? Tight and toned upper arms? A rounded rear with that cute cheek dimple? All these are goals that can be achieved through the *Lower Body Solution.*

The routines presented in this book break with traditional body-building routines prescribed by most personal trainers. For instance, most women are not terribly interested in developing all of the small muscles of the biceps, upper back and shoulders. Therefore, instead of many isolation exercises for these muscles, the program uses compound movements, such as pull-ups, push-ups, pulldowns and dips. The muscular development from such exercises is more smooth and flowing, rather than the hard, angular development some bodybuilders seek.

Women tend to carry fat, and lack muscle tone, on the back of their arms (the triceps region), so additional triceps work is interspersed throughout the workouts. Since the triceps tend to be a "weak link" in a woman's upper body, additional strengthening is necessary to get the full benefits from upper body exercises.

The lower body is composed of large, powerful muscles. Training these muscles is key to achieving the increased caloric expenditure most women want. Therefore, logically, the program concentrates on lower body exercise. To prevent these muscles from growing overly large—and to actually help diminish their size—a very high frequency of lower body training is used. As explained previously, this is the same method that ice skaters and dancers use to retain muscular strength but stay small in size. The lower body is where the emphasis is put.

Chest training is given a high degree of importance in conventional routines because the chest is an important muscle group for a man to develop. Breasts, not chests, are the showy part of a woman's upper front torso. Unfortunately, chest training does little to enhance the breasts. It is not true that chest training can lift the breasts, remove stretch marks or cause the breasts to decrease in size. Breasts are composed of fat, not muscle, and are thus unaffected by weight training. Weight training will affect the underlying muscle, which can add depth to the upper chest. Weight training does contribute to an overall loss of body fat, which in turn may decrease the size of the breasts since they are composed of fat. Chest training should be given a moderate priority in a woman's routine, much the same as the arms, back and shoulders.

The *Lower Body Solution* concentrates on the large muscles of the body for maximum calories burned; however, it doesn't ignore the smaller muscles. While working these smaller muscles may do little to increase calories burned, they are absolutely essential to proper posture and the overall health of your back. Therefore, postural exercises and stretching are a part of the exercise routines.

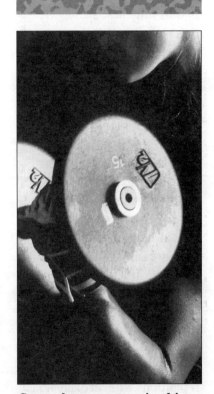

Several parameters in this program are specifically manipulated so that you will not build the muscle size associated with female bodybuilders. Exertion and effort are rewarded in this program with a loss of fat, not with muscle size.

Development of the small muscles that stabilize the upper torso has as much to do with back training as it does with abdominal training.

The Lower Body Intensity Zone

Just as there is an ideal heart rate intensity in aerobic exercise, there is an ideal weight intensity for women who weight train for weight loss. Every weight training exercise will prescribe a number of repetitions. That number is usually between eight and fifteen. We'll use ten as an example in the following explanation of the proper weight intensity zone.

If you are striving to perform ten repetitions, you ideally need to find a weight that allows you to perform the first six repetitions easily, the seventh and eighth with a little effort, and the ninth and tenth with more effort. You should never use a weight that requires you to sacrifice form, or "cheat", to complete the tenth repetition. If your exercise prescription says to perform ten reps for three sets, you should never use a weight that doesn't allow you to complete at least ten of the repetitions in the first set, nine of the repetitions in the second set, and eight of the repetitions in the third set. Further, you need to add more weight if you can complete all your repetitions with virtually no effort.

What I've just described puts your weight training in a zone that can effectively contribute to lean body mass but will not promote large muscle growth. The *Lower Body Solution* is different from other weight training programs in that it keeps you at 65 to 75 percent of your maximal exertion level. To build large muscle you must train at 80 to 100 percent of your maximal ability. However, training at less than 65 percent of your maximal ability does nothing to build the muscle tone necessary to increase your metabolism and help you control your weight once and for all. So it is extremely important that you find the 65 to 75 percent fat-burning intensity level at which you should lift weights.

While all this may seem confusing, as you begin this program you'll discover very quickly what weight you should be lifting. This may change depending on the day—we all have high-energy/strong days and low-energy/weak days. Each day you perform a weightlifting routine, adjust your weight according to how you are feeling that day.

This program moves through stages. At times, your weight training will seem very easy. Other times it takes a lot of effort and creates a lactic acid "burn" in your legs, similar to how you feel when you "hit the wall" while running. I'll warn you when those stages occur in the program, but consider that when you have a tough day that takes extra effort, there is an easy day that follows!

> *Just as there is an ideal heart rate intensity in aerobic exercise, there is an ideal weight intensity for women who weight train for weight loss.*

What If I'm Sore?

You'll notice as you progress through this program that there may be some slight muscle soreness. This is normal and you should not only accept it, but welcome the feeling! Muscle soreness will occur in varying degrees as your body adjusts to the routine. It is a signal that your body is building muscle tone, which in turn increases your metabolism for better fat-burning efficiency.

However, if you become so sore that you can't go about your daily activities, go back and reread the discussion on intensity levels. This program is designed to cause some muscle soreness, but never debilitating soreness. Severe muscle soreness should be treated with rest and warm baths, followed by walking or another form of easy stretching exercise. Aspirin may also provide some relief.

I Can Do Anything (For One More Set)

One thing that helps me and my clients get through the tough days is to look at each set of exercises as an end in themselves. "I can do anything for just one more set!" has gotten us through thousands of third sets. Also, remember that when it comes to fat loss, often it's that third set that really counts. And when cardio starts to look like the endless mile, check your monitor and say to yourself, "I can do anything for fifteen (or ten or five) more minutes."

One of the marvelous things about weight training is that it gives you instant milestones. You may do aerobic classes for three weeks without seeing any results, but when you begin weight training you will see changes in your strength immediately—some going up, some down. Each weight training workout will give you immediate feedback, and you will see a dramatic change in your strength and range of motion in just two weeks—yes, dramatic! Each of these increments is a step toward better health and fitness, and a step toward lifelong weight control. When you do reach the "melting" weeks of the program, you'll enjoy a loss of pounds like you've never imagined!

The Routine

*H*ere's what you've been waiting for: **THE ROUTINE!**

The *Lower Body Solution* is a four-to-seven-month program that can be adapted into a program for life. Depending on your personal circumstances, you will begin the program at level one, level two or level three.

The *Lower Body Solution* is designed to attack the most stubborn female fat. Fat is most often lost in reverse of the way it is gained. Therefore, if you have always had fat thighs, your thighs will unfortunately be the last area where you will see radical changes. That's the bad news. The good news is that in the process you will have transformed your body from a fat-collecting machine to a fat-burning machine. This will help make keeping the weight off easier.

To Begin

The *Lower Body Solution* has three levels:

Level One: Baseline strength, flexibility and muscular endurance development (nine weeks)

Level Two: Warm-up workouts for high-frequency exercise (three weeks)

Level Three: Shrink the thighs, hips, lower belly and decrease overall body fat (16 weeks)

Find Your Level

Find the category that best describes your present condition and goals to identify your starting level:

Level One:
- Never exercised before
- Haven't exercised regularly for more than a year
- Had a baby less than three months ago
- Have chronic back and/or knee injuries
- Trying to lose 50 or more pounds
- Over 60 years old

Level Two:
- Have been an active exerciser, but not for the past several months
- Trying to lose fewer than 30 pounds, but otherwise in good health

Level Three:
- Trying to lose fewer than 15 pounds, mostly in the lower body, and
- Exercise regularly, and in good health

Repeating Level Three

Once you have completed level three, you can repeat it as many times as you like—for years if you want!

Of course, by the time you've completed level three you will be quite familiar with your body and the workouts as well. Therefore, I'd suggest you begin to customize the routine to your goals. You may want to expand by a week or even two some of the routines that you found particularly enjoyable and/or result-producing. You may want to add some extra work for your shoulders (to make your waist appear smaller) or your abdominals (see Chapter 16 for Advanced Exercises). Be creative! Just make certain you avoid maximum intensities in both the aerobic and weight training portions of the program, and that you change your routine at least every three weeks.

LBS Basic Training Tenets

The *Lower Body Solution* uses a variety of training techniques to produce the changes you want to see. You may find the cardio weeks to be the most fun and fulfilling. Or, you may find the strength-building phases or fat-burning weeks give you the most pleasure and best results. We are all different, and the workouts that may be your favorites may change according to the season as well. I know that I don't like long cardio in the summer because it's too hot. On the other hand, gloomy winter weather can put a damper on my strength-building workouts, which are my personal favorites.

There are bound to be one or two workouts that you find difficult. Just remind yourself that it's only for a few weeks (sometimes only days). "You can do anything for three days!" is what I like to tell my clients. The beauty of the *Lower Body Solution* is that it is always changing, and it is always challenging your body. Further, for each of the really grueling workouts, there is always an easy workout that follows.

I understand that time constraints, busy health clubs and equipment limitations may force you to slightly alter some of the workouts. When this occurs, remember some of the basic "rules" of the *Lower Body Solution*:

- Compound (more than one muscle group) exercise is preferred to isolation (one muscle group) exercise.
- Freeweight exercises are preferred to machines.
- Move from one muscle group to another; do not perform all the exercises for one muscle group consecutively.
- Do not perform the exact same exercise, in the same set and rep pattern, two days in a row (exceptions are some abdominal, posture and stretching exercises).
- The periods of rest between sets and between exercises gradually decrease in the workouts until optimal rest times are achieved.

How Much Time Does It Really Take?

One magazine study found that most women are only willing to spend 20 minutes a day exercising, three days a week. I believe there is some truth to that. I know for sure that many women simply don't have the time to spend an hour at the health club six days a week. Therefore, the *Lower Body Solution* is set up for maximum flexibility.

The *Lower Body Solution* takes 30-60 minutes per routine and can be performed up to six days a week. In the level three workouts you have three mandatory days and three optional days. Some routines can be performed at home. Those who can only do the program three times a week can still enjoy excellent results, but the results are slower in coming. If you have more time, work out more days. The results will be more gratifying if you spend more time with the program.

If you miss days, just keep plugging along. The program assumes that you won't be able to work out six days a week, every week. If you can only get in the three mandatory days and one home day, fine! Even if you only get in the three mandatory days, it's fine (but I suggest you reread Chapter 7, You're Kidding! Me? Work Out Six Days a Week to Slim My Thighs?) If you miss a week of training, or are only able to get in one

workout that week, repeat the week—don't skip to the next week or the next workout. If you miss two weeks, just pick up at the first week missed. However, if you miss three weeks, you don't pass Go and you do have to start the level three workouts from the beginning again. The workouts are designed to build upon each other, and skipping weeks will not provide you with the optimal fat-burning stimuli.

Each workout you complete moves your body a notch closer to becoming a fat-burning machine. Anyone who has been in shape can tell you that the benefits from exercise stick with you long after the exercise has been performed. Muscle has memory, and even if you miss two or three weeks, when you get back on the program your body will catch up at a much faster rate than if you had never exercised before.

Remember, missing a workout is not going to cause you to fall off the program. It is just going to slow your progress. Ask yourself just how badly you want to get in shape. If you want it badly enough, you won't miss many workouts. Also, as the pounds drop off and your conditioning improves, you'll find that your discipline and energy level improve as well.

Day-by-Day Instruction

Each weekly training program begins with an explanation of what to expect that week. Your workouts are listed day by day, with room for you to keep track of your workout days and weights lifted. For complete explanations and photos of each of the exercises used, refer to the Exercise Index at the back of this book.

If you have a workout partner, great! I've always enjoyed working out with a friend. If you don't have a partner, bring this book along. Refer back to the introduction of each routine as you perform it, and perhaps add some of your own comments to those of myself and my clients. Think of this book as your "partner."

Okay partner, let's begin.

Lower Body Solution Level One

This nine-week program will get you familiar with weight training. It will teach you some of the core exercises, plus several isolation exercises for your abdominals and lower back to improve your posture, and increase your muscular endurance to prepare you for the more advanced workouts. It begins very slow, starting with just one set per exercise, and builds each week. It is paced so that each week you will build muscle strength and endurance. For a beginner, it is the healthiest thing you can do for your body; however, it is not designed to produce dramatic weight loss.

Even if you have been athletic all your life, if you fall into one or more of the level one criteria, you need to follow this routine as it is written, one step at a time. Jumping ahead before you are ready will not lead to optimal weight loss. Progressing too quickly can also lead to uncomfortable and unnecessary muscular soreness.

Level One

You're ready to do it! This week you're going to get familiar with some of the exercises and equipment in the health club. Don't be afraid to ask the trainers if you have a question—they are there to help!

If this is your first time ever lifting weights, go back and reread Chapter 11, First-Time Lifters, before you go into the health club. Make sure you do not overdo anything this first week. You will most likely have to adjust the weights on the machines a few times to find a comfortable weight for your first set. Consider this your "preview" week—it's just to familiarize your muscles with the exercises; you won't be setting any world records!

For you eager-beavers, please don't be tempted to do more—there's lots more later, so don't rush it! Also, although only two workouts are considered mandatory, three are optimal and would increase your fat-burning results by one-third!

Be sure to write down the amount of weight you use next to each of the exercises. Since this workout is just a trial run, experiment with finding a weight that causes just a little strain (not a lot, and certainly not an all-out effort!) to complete the required repetitions. Don't worry if it takes three or four attempts to find the right weight. It gets easier each workout.

Don't forget to stretch following your workouts or in the evenings. A basic lower-body stretching program is presented in Chapter 14.

Okay, let's get started!

Week Beginning:

_____

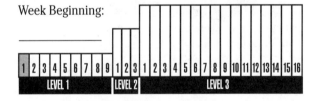

Level One, Week 1

Frequency: Two nonconsecutive days
Rest between sets: Two minutes (yes, wait an entire two minutes!)
Rest between exercises: At least 90 seconds; not more than three minutes
Tempo: For lower-body exercises, lower the weight in four seconds and lift in two seconds.

For upper-body exercises, lower the weight in three seconds and lift in two seconds.
Comments: You only perform one set of each weight training exercise and 10 minutes of cardio, so these workouts will be very brief (no more than 30 minutes). Also, when you're ready to perform a weight training exercise, start with a light resistance and work your way up to a weight that causes a slight exertion.

You will start this routine with the pelvic tilt. Read the full explanation of how to perform this very small movement. Although it's hard to believe, shifting your pelvis less than two inches to perform this movement is 200 times more effective at toning your lower abdominals than performing a sit-up! The movement takes several workout sessions to master, and you may not feel much at all the first few weeks. Give it time. It works!

Weights		Week 1, Workouts 1 and 2	Reps/Sets
—	—	Pelvic Tilt	10x1
—	—	Lunge, Stationary	10x1
—	—	(opt. Leg Extension	10x1)†
—	—	Lateral Raise	8x1
—	—	Leg Curl, Seated	10x1
—	—	One-Arm Row, Dumbbell	8x1
—	—	Prone Cobra	10x1
—	—	Stationary Bicycle	10 minutes, at 5-7 PRE*

†Optional Exercise
*Perceived Rate of Exertion (for a full explanation, see Chapter 10)

Comments: _____

_____

_____

Week Beginning:

_____

Level One, Week 2
Frequency: Two nonconsecutive days.
Rest Between Sets: Two minutes
Rest Between Exercises: 90 seconds to three minutes
Tempo: For lower-body exercises, lower the weight in four seconds and lift in two seconds. For upper-body exercises, lower the weight in three seconds and lift in two seconds.

Comments: Ready, set and go to the health club for your first real workout. It's the same set of exercises from the week before, except you're now going to perform two sets for most of the weight training exercises.

You should be familiar with the weights to use and will probably run through this workout more smoothly than last week. This week you may actually start to discover some muscles you never even knew you had!

Weights	Week 2, Workouts 1 and 2	
__ __	Pelvic Tilt	10x1
__ __	Lunge, Stationary	10x2
__ __	(opt. Leg Press, Horizontal	10x2)
__ __	Lateral Raise	8x2
__ __	Leg Curl, Seated	10x2
__ __	One-Arm Row, Dumbbell	8x2
__ __	Prone Cobra	10x1
__ __	Stationary Bicycle	12 minutes, at 5-7 PRE

Comments: _____

_____

_____

Week Beginning: _____

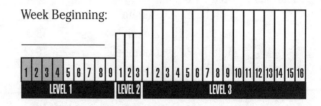

Level One, Week 3

Frequency: Two nonconsecutive days; three nonconsecutive days if you have the energy!

Rest Between Sets: Two minutes

Rest Between Exercises: 90 seconds to three minutes

Tempo: For lower-body exercises, lower the weight in four seconds and lift in two seconds. For upper-body exercises, lower the weight in three seconds and lift in two seconds.

Comments: You should be feeling confident on these exercises and may want to increase the weights just a little bit. This week you will begin doing three sets on some of the movements and also will become familiar with some new exercises. You have an optional day this week, and I heartily suggest you try to work it in.

Have you taken all your beginning measurements and weighed yourself? If not, be sure to do so this week. Then check every couple of weeks and note your progress. How about progress on the lifts? Have you increased several of your weights? You should already be feeling stronger.

Weights	Week 3, Workouts 1 and 2	
__ __	Pelvic Tilt	10x1
__ __	Lunge, Stationary	10x3
__ __	Biceps Curl with Shoulder Press	8x3
__ __	(opt. Lateral Raise	8x3)

__ __	Leg Curl, Seated	10x3
__ __	One-Arm Row, Dumbbell	8x3
__ __	Prone Cobra	10x1
__ __	Stationary Bicycle	15 minutes, at 5-7 PRE

Weights	Week 3, Workout 3 (Optional)	
__ __	Abdominal Crunch	10x1
__ __	Lunge, Reverse	10x3
__ __	(opt. Leg Press, Inclined	10x3)
__ __	Lateral Raise	8x3
__ __	Triceps Pressdown	10x3
__ __	Pulldown to Chest	8x3
__ __	Prone Cobra	10x1
__ __	Stationary Bicycle	15 minutes, at 5-7 PRE

Comments: _____

_____

_____

Week Beginning: _____

Level One, Week 4

Frequency: Two nonconsecutive days; three nonconsecutive days if you have the energy!

Rest Between Sets: 90 seconds

Rest Between Exercises: One to two minutes

Tempo: For lower-body exercises, lower the weight in four seconds and lift in two seconds. For upper-body exercises, lower the weight in three seconds and lift in two seconds.

Comments: Congratulations! You are ready to begin the first week of a three-week segment designed to increase your base level of strength and adjust your metabolism for maximum fat-burning. For this purpose we have shortened the time between your exercise sets.

I know you were feeling confident on last week's exercises, but this week is a whole new ballgame. You may need two or three starts to find the right poundages again. Be sure to write them down to keep track for your next workout. You'll be performing these exercises for a total of three weeks.

Remember, if you feel any discomfort, lengthen the time between sets or go back and repeat weeks 2 and

3. If you're feeling really great, don't change the rest times or tempo, but add a third nonconsecutive day to the week!

For this week, you will only perform two sets of each of the major weight training exercises, but you'll increase to three sets next week. This reduced level will help prevent muscle soreness. Also, note that the amount of time between exercises has been reduced.

Weights	Week 4, Workout 1 (Mandatory)	
__ __	Reverse Crunch	12x1
__ __	Squat, Ballet	12x2
__ __	Leg Press, Horizontal	12x2
__ __	Military Press, Dumbbells	10x2
__ __	Leg Curl, Prone	12x2
__ __	Rowing Machine, Seated	10x2
__ __	Horse Stance	3 reps, hold 10 seconds, 1 set
__ __	Treadmill	20 minutes, at 5-7 PRE

Weights	Week 4, Workout 2 (Mandatory)	
__ __	Reverse Crunch	12x1
__ __	Squat, Dumbbells	12x2
__ __	(opt. Petersen Step-up	12x2)
__ __	Leg Press, Horizontal	12x2
__ __	Military Press, Dumbbells	10x2
__ __	(opt. Lateral Raise	10x2)
__ __	Leg Curl, Prone	12x2
__ __	Rowing Machine, Seated	10x2
__ __	Horse Stance	3 reps, hold 10 seconds, 1 set
__ __	Treadmill	20 minutes, at 5-7 PRE

Weights	Week 4, Workout 3 (Optional)	
__ __	Reverse Crunch	12x1
__ __	Squat, Dumbbells	12x2
__ __	(opt. Leg Extension	12x2)
__ __	Leg Press, Horizontal	12x2
__ __	Military Press, Dumbbells	10x2
__ __	(opt. Lateral Raise	10x2)
__ __	Leg Curl, Prone	12x2
__ __	Rowing Machine, Seated	10x2
__ __	Horse Stance	3 reps, hold 10 seconds, 1 set
__ __	Treadmill	20 minutes, at 5-7 PRE

Comments: _____

_____

_____

Week Beginning:

_____

1 2 3 4 5 6 7 8 9	1 2 3	1	2 3 4 5 6 7 8 9 10 11 12 13 14 15 16
LEVEL 1	LEVEL 2		LEVEL 3

Level One, Week 5

Frequency: The first two workouts should be performed on nonconsecutive days; the third optional routine can be performed anytime, but not on the same day as the first two!

Rest Between Sets: 90 seconds

Rest Between Exercises: One to two minutes

Tempo: For lower-body exercises, lower the weight in four seconds and lift in two seconds. For upper-body exercises, lower the weight in three seconds and lift in two seconds.

Comments: If you haven't already, now is a good time to take your measurements and start recording your bodyweight (in the morning, no clothes!). The biggest changes right now will be in your conditioning, but you want those "before" measurements and weight recorded to see your weight loss progress, which is right around the corner!

Note that you are back up to three sets of each of the major weight training exercises. As you might have suspected, the first exercise is always an abdominal exercise performed for one set as a warm-up. Additional work for the abdominals, at a much greater effort level, is provided in level two and level three in the home workouts.

If you are not seeing the overall weight loss you want, try increasing your cardio times or adding some of the extra-burn workouts outlined in Chapter 6.

Weights	Week 5, Workout 1 (Mandatory)	
__ __	Reverse Crunch	12x1
__ __	Squat, Ballet	12x3
__ __	(opt. Peterson Step-Up	12x3)
__ __	Leg Press, Horizontal	12x3
__ __	Military Press, Dumbbells	10x3
__ __	(opt. Lateral Raise	10x3)
__ __	Leg Curl, Prone	12x3
__ __	Rowing Machine, Seated	10x3
__ __	Horse Stance	3 reps, hold 10 seconds, 1 set
__ __	Treadmill	20 minutes, at 5-7 PRE

Weights	Week 5, Workout 2 (Mandatory)	
__ __	Reverse Crunch	12x1
__ __	Squat, Dumbbells	12x3
__ __	(opt. Lunge, Reverse	12x3)
__ __	Leg Press, Horizontal	12x3

Weights			
__	__	Military Press, Dumbbells	10x3
__	__	(opt. Lateral Raise	10x3)
__	__	Leg Curl, Prone	12x3
__	__	Rowing Machine, Seated	10x3
__	__	Horse Stance	3 reps,
			hold 10 seconds, 1 set
__	__	Treadmill	20 minutes, at 5-7 PRE

Weights   **Week 5, Workout 3 (Optional)**

__	__	Pelvic Tilt	15x1
__	__	Lunge, Stationary	10x3
__	__	Biceps Curl with Shoulder Press	10x3
__	__	(opt. Biceps Curl, Dumbbells	10x3)
__	__	Leg Curl, Seated	10x3
__	__	One-Arm Row, Dumbbell	10x3
__	__	Prone Cobra	10x1
__	__	Stationary Bicycle 20 minutes, at 5-7 PRE	

Comments: _____

_____

_____

Week Beginning:

_____

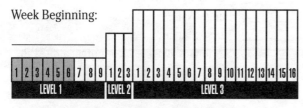

Level One, Week 6

Frequency: Two nonconsecutive days; three nonconsecutive days if you have the energy!

Rest Between Sets: 90 seconds

Rest Between Exercises: One to two minutes

Tempo: For lower-body exercises, lower the weight in four seconds and lift in two seconds. For upper-body exercises, lower the weight in three seconds and lift in two seconds.

Comments: At this point you should be noticing muscles you never knew you had before! You should also be sleeping better and feeling better. The amount of exercise you have completed up to this point has already increased your overall strength levels, and now that strength will become increasingly apparent. When you put the groceries away or shift objects from one storage cabinet to another, you will start to notice that even these small tasks are getting easier. Heck, getting up out of a chair is taking 35 percent less effort, according to those folks who study such mundane things! And you ain't seen nothin' yet!

Weights   **Week 6, Workout 1 (Mandatory)**

__	__	Reverse Crunch	12x1
__	__	Squat, Dumbbells	12x3
__	__	(opt. Peterson Step-Up	12x3)
__	__	Leg Press, Horizontal	12x3
__	__	Military Press, Dumbbells	10x3
__	__	(opt. Lateral Raise	10x3)
__	__	Leg Curl, Prone	12x3
__	__	Rowing Machine, Seated	10x3
__	__	Horse Stance	3 reps,
			hold 10 seconds, 1 set
__	__	Treadmill	20 minutes, at 5-7 PRE

Weights   **Week 6, Workout 2 (Mandatory)**

__	__	Reverse Crunch	12x1
__	__	Squat, Dumbbells	12x3
__	__	(opt. Leg Extension	12x3)
__	__	Leg Press, Horizontal	12x3
__	__	Military Press, Dumbbells	10x3
__	__	(opt. Bench Press, Machine	10x3)
__	__	Leg Curl, Prone	12x3
__	__	Rowing Machine, Seated	10x3
__	__	Horse Stance	3 reps,
			hold 10 seconds, 1 set
__	__	Treadmill	20 minutes, at 5-7 PRE

Weights   **Week 6, Workout 3 (Optional)**

__	__	Reverse Crunch	12x1
__	__	Squat, Dumbbells	12x3
__	__	(opt. Peterson Step-Up	12x3)
__	__	Leg Press, Horizontal	12x3
__	__	Military Press, Dumbbells	10x3
__	__	(opt. Lateral Raise	10x3)
__	__	Leg Curl, Prone	12x3
__	__	Rowing Machine, Seated	10x3
__	__	Horse Stance	3 reps,
			hold 10 seconds, 1 set
__	__	Treadmill	20 minutes, at 5-7 PRE

Comments: _____

_____

_____

Week Beginning:

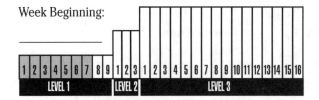

_____

Level One, Week 7

Frequency: The first two workouts should be performed on nonconsecutive days; the third optional routine can be performed anytime, but not on the same day as either of the the first two!

Rest Between Sets: 60 seconds

Rest Between Exercises: One to two minutes

Tempo: For lower-body exercises, lower the weight in four seconds and lift in two seconds. For upper-body exercises, lower the weight in three seconds and lift in two seconds.

Comments: Time to look back at how far we've come! You're about to complete the sixth week of your base-level conditioning. Do you remember the first few days of the routine, when the weights, the effort, the exercises and the machines all seemed strange and perhaps a bit intimidating?

At this point you should be feeling all the positive confidence-boosters that come along with weight training. You have taken a major, positive step in improving both your muscular strength and your endurance. You're not sitting around letting your body take its own course of direction-you are directing that course and making huge strides toward building a body that you will be proud of.

I know many of you may not have seen the dramatic weight loss you're ultimately looking for, but remember your level one workouts are intended to build baseline strength and muscular endurance! The fat-burning comes in just a few short weeks. Hang in there; it's all scientifically mapped out to ensure your greatest success.

There are several new and exciting exercises introduced this week. Check out the descriptions in the Exercise Index. This is the first week you'll begin doing a Lunge, Front. For anyone with knee problems, please use the Lunge, Reverse if you experience any discomfort. You'll also be doing your first "combination" movement, the Biceps Curl with Shoulder Press. This is a great exercise for shaping up the upper arms.

Weights	Week 7, Workout 1 (Mandatory)	
__ __	Cross Crunch	15x1
__ __	Lunge, Front	15x2
__ __	(opt. Lunge, Reverse	15x2)
__ __	Leg Press, Horizontal	15x2
__ __	Biceps Curl with Shoulder Press	10x3
__ __	(opt. Biceps Curl, Dumbbells	10x3)
__ __	Leg Curl, Seated	15x2
__ __	One-Arm Row, Dumbbell	10x2
__ __	Prone Cobra	15x1
__ __	Treadmill	20 minutes, at 6-8 PRE

Weights Week 7, Workout 2 (Mandatory)

__ __	Cross Crunch	15x1
__ __	Lunge, Front	15x2
__ __	(opt. Lunge, Reverse	15x2)
__ __	Leg Press, Horizontal	15x2
__ __	Biceps Curl with Shoulder Press	10x3
__ __	(opt. Bench Press, Machine)	
__ __	Leg Curl, Seated	15x2
__ __	One-Arm Row, Dumbbell	10x2
__ __	Prone Cobra	15x1
__ __	Treadmill	20 minutes, at 6-8 PRE

Weights Week 7, Workout 3 (Optional)

__ __	Abdominal Crunch	15x2
__ __	Lunge, Front	12x3
__ __	(opt. Lunge, Reverse	12x3)
__ __	Lateral Raise	10x2
__ __	Leg Extension	10x3
__ __	Triceps Pressdown	10x3
__ __	Pulldown to Chest	10x3
__ __	Lunge Walk	2 minutes
__ __	Horse Stance	10x1
__ __	Stationary Bicycle 25 minutes, at 5-7 PRE	

Comments: _____

_____

_____

Week Beginning:

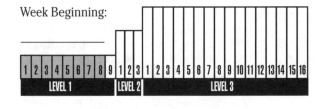

_____

Level One, Week 8

Frequency: The first two workouts should be performed on nonconsecutive days; the third optional routine can be performed anytime, but not on the same day as either of the first two!

Rest Between Sets: 60 seconds

Rest Between Exercises: One to two minutes

Tempo: For lower-body exercises, lower the weight in four seconds and lift in two seconds. For upper-body exercises, lower the weight in three seconds and lift in two seconds.

Comments: Welcome to the world of weights! You're going to notice the next three weeks will take a bit more effort than the previous weeks, but you've built yourself up for it and you're ready. This is where the real fun begins!

Because I've shortened the rest time between sets (from 90 to 60 seconds), for this week I'm recommending that you perform only two sets of each of the major weight training exercises. Next week you'll be back up to three sets. This adjustment will help prevent muscle soreness. Get in there, and get with it. What's coming around the corner is something you've probably desired for quite some time—a major, positive change in your body!

Weights	Week 8, Workout 1 (Mandatory)	
__ __	Cross Crunch	15x1
__ __	Lunge, Reverse	15x3
__ __	Leg Press, Horizontal	15x3
__ __	Lateral Raise	12x3
__ __	Leg Curl, Seated	15x3
__ __	One-Arm Row, Dumbbell	12x3
__ __	Prone Cobra	15x1
__ __	Treadmill	20 minutes, at 6-8 PRE

Weights	Week 8, Workout 2 (Mandatory)	
__ __	Cross Crunch	15x1
__ __	Lunge, Reverse	15x3
__ __	Leg Press, Horizontal	15x3
__ __	Lateral Raise	12x3
__ __	Leg Curl, Seated	15x3
__ __	One-Arm Row, Dumbbell	12x3
__ __	Prone Cobra	15x1
__ __	Treadmill	20 minutes, at 6-8 PRE

Weights	Week 8, Workout 3 (Optional)	
__ __	Abdominal Crunch	15x2
__ __	Lunge, Front	12x3
__ __	Lateral Raise	10x2
__ __	Leg Extension	10x3
__ __	Triceps Pressdown	10x3
__ __	Pulldown to Chest	10x3
__ __	Lunge Walk	2 minutes
__ __	Horse Stance	10x1
__ __	Stationary Bicycle	25 minutes, at 5-7 PRE

Comments: _____

_____

_____

Week Beginning:

Level One, Week 9

Frequency: The first two workouts should be performed on nonconsecutive days; the third optional routine can be performed anytime, but not on the same day as either of the first two!

Rest Between Sets: 60 seconds

Rest Between Exercises: One to two minutes

Tempo: For lower-body exercises, lower the weight in four seconds and lift in two seconds. For upper-body exercises, lower the weight in three seconds and lift in two seconds.

Comments: Yes! You have nearly completed the level one workout. At this point, I suspect some of you are ready for your first powerlifting meet! Well, maybe not. But isn't weight training a great new way to exercise? Have you found that it's easier lugging those groceries home? How about your general energy level or your self-confidence now that you've worked on and gained new muscular strength and endurance? Take a few moments to congratulate yourself in getting your body on track for the workouts to come.

You're only one week away from the level two workouts, which will be a dramatic change from these past weeks. Feel a little soreness in your legs and chest? Warm baths help, and feel great even if you're not sore!

Keep track of your poundages—you may have to experiment once or twice since you're using an entirely new routine of exercises this week. And keep track of your measurements and weight as well. You should be seeing a positive change!

Weights	Week 9, Workout 1 (Mandatory)	
__ __	Cross Crunch	15x1
__ __	Lunge, Stationary	15x3
__ __	Leg Press, Horizontal	15x3
__ __	Lateral Raise	12x3
__ __	Leg Curl, Seated	15x3
__ __	One-Arm Row, Dumbbell	12x3
__ __	Prone Cobra	15x1
__ __	Treadmill	20 minutes, at 6-8 PRE

Weights | **Week 9, Workout 2 (Mandatory)** |
--- | --- | ---
__ __ | Cross Crunch | 15x1
__ __ | Lunge, Stationary | 15x3
__ __ | Leg Press, Horizontal | 15x3
__ __ | Lateral Raise | 12x3
__ __ | Leg Curl, Seated | 15x3
__ __ | One-Arm Row, Dumbbell | 12x3
__ __ | Prone Cobra | 15x1
__ __ | Treadmill | 20 minutes, at 6-8 PRE

Weights | **Week 9, Workout 3 (Optional)** |
--- | --- | ---
__ __ | Abdominal Crunch | 15x2
__ __ | Lunge, Front | 12x3
__ __ | Lateral Raise | 10x2
__ __ | Leg Extension | 10x3
__ __ | Triceps Pressdown | 10x3
__ __ | Pulldown to Chest | 10x3
__ __ | Lunge Walk | 2 minutes
__ __ | (opt. Lunge, Stationary | 12x3)
__ __ | Horse Stance | 10x1
__ __ | Stationary Bicycle | 25 minutes, at 5-7 PRE

Comments: _____

_____

_____

Level Two Workouts

Welcome to level two! If you've worked your way up from level one I bet you have some favorite exercises now. How about least favorite? It seems the exercises you're weakest on are usually the least favorite, but probably the most beneficial to you. One of the great things about the *Lower Body Solution* is that it is constantly changing, always giving you a new workout to follow and keeping your body challenged by what's coming next. That's the secret to seeing continual results from weight training.

We all know that it's going to take some effort to get in shape and stay that way. Still, it's not reasonable to think that we can push ourselves every workout, every week. That's why these programs will shift in emphasis. You never have to endure the really tough workouts for more than three weeks, and most of the time even less!

If you've already begun to see a loss in weight and/or inches, great. If not, consider the fact that an overweight individual who exercises on a program such as this is healthier than an overweight individual who doesn't exercise. You need to be as aware of your physical health as you are of your weight. Congratulate

yourself on the milestones you're making in the health club with each new exercise you learn and each increase in weight you lift.

If you are just joining the *Lower Body Solution* at level two, welcome! The next three weeks will be spent in a routine designed to prepare your lower body for the level three workouts to come.

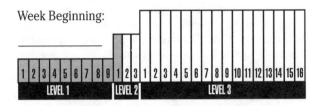

Week Beginning:

Level Two, Week One

Frequency: Three days in the health club; a fourth optional day at home

Rest Between Sets: 60 seconds

Rest Between Exercises: 45 seconds to two minutes

Tempo: For lower-body exercises, lower the weight in four seconds and lift in two seconds. For upper-body exercises, lower the weight in three seconds and lift in two seconds.

Comments: As in the workouts in level one, the first exercise in level two is always an abdominal exercise performed for just one set. It's used as a warm-up. This first week you are performing only two sets for most of the major exercises. Take it easy; there's much more to come!

The next three weeks are designed to get you familiar with the exercises and routines and also to prepare you for the high-frequency workouts to come. Don't go all out just yet—ease into this program and read the exercise descriptions carefully so you can master each of the moves with precision. The real work is yet to come; these three weeks are still on the upside of the learning curve.

Perform these workouts in the order listed and make sure you rest the proper time between sets and exercises. Every small nuance in this routine is carefully planned to set the stage for major fat reduction in future workouts.

Weights	**Week 1, Workout 1 (Mandatory)**	**Reps/Sets**
__ __	Pelvic Tilt	15x1
__ __	Cross Crunch	15x1
__ __	Lunge, Front	15x2
__ __	Petersen Step-Up	15x2
__ __	Military Press, Dumbbells	12x2
__ __	Leg Curl, Prone	15x2
__ __	One-Arm Row, Dumbbell	12x2

—	—	Abduction, Multi-Hip Machine	15x2
—	—	Pec Dec	12x2
—	—	Triceps Pressdown	12x2
—	—	Calf Raise, Standing	15x2
—	—	Prone Cobra	15x1
—	—	Treadmill	25 minutes, at 5-7 PRE

Weights — Week 1, Workout 2 (Mandatory)

—	—	Abdominal Crunch	15x2
—	—	Pulldown to Chest	12x2
—	—	Leg Press, Horizontal	12x2
—	—	Lateral Raise	12x2
—	—	Adduction, Multi-Hip Machine	15x3
—	—	Bench Press, Incline Machine	10x2
—	—	Triceps Pressdown	12x2
—	—	Leg Extension	12x2
—	—	Biceps Curl, Dumbbells	10x2
—	—	Stairclimber	10 minutes, at 5-7 PRE
—	—	Treadmill	15 minutes, at 5-7 PRE

Weights — Week 1, Workout 3 (Mandatory)

—	—	Pelvic Tilt	15x1
—	—	Cross Crunch	15x1
—	—	Lunge, Front	15x2
—	—	Peterson Step-Up	15x2
—	—	Military Press, Dumbbells	12x2
—	—	Leg Curl, Prone	15x2
—	—	One-Arm Row, Dumbbell	12x2
—	—	Abduction, Multi-Hip	15x2
—	—	Pec Dec	12x2
—	—	Triceps Pressdown	12x2
—	—	Calf Raise, Standing	15x2
—	—	Prone Cobra	15x1
—	—	Treadmill	25 minutes, at 5-7 PRE

Wts. — Week 1, Workout 4 (Home, Optional)

—	—	Lunge, Reverse	8x4
—	—	Push-Up	12x2
—	—	Squat, Ballet	10x3
—	—	Lunge, Stationary	10x3
—	—	Chair Dip	10x3
—	—	Lunge, Front	10x3

Comments: _____

_____

_____

*PRE - Perceived Rate of Exertion (see Ch. 10)

Week Beginning:

Level Two, Week 2

Frequency: Three days in the health club; one day at home

Rest Between Sets: 60 seconds

Rest Between Exercises: 45 seconds to two minutes

Tempo: For lower-body exercises, lower the weight in four seconds and lift in two seconds. For upper-body exercises, lower the weight in three seconds and lift in two seconds.

Comments: Getting a little idea of why I said this isn't like any other weight training program? Consistency is the key; but the only real consistency is that you work out every week. That's why this program works for so many different types of people: old, young, really overweight, moderately overweight. It's as different as all the types of people it works for!

This week you're doing three sets of the major exercises. If it's taking a long time to get through the workouts, don't worry. We'll be trimming minutes off your rest times in the next few weeks, and as you become more familiar with each of the exercises, you'll be moving through them a bit quicker. Next week you'll increase the intensity of the cardio, moving from a PRE (perceived rate of exertion) level of 5-7 to 6-8. That's where we're going to start seeing some real fat-burning!

Weights — Week 2, Workout 1 (Mandatory)

—	—	Pelvic Tilt	15x1
—	—	Cross Crunch	15x1
—	—	Lunge, Front	15x2
—	—	Peterson Step-Up	15x2
—	—	Military Press, Dumbbells	12x2
—	—	Leg Curl, Prone	15x2
—	—	One-Arm Row, Dumbbell	12x2
—	—	Abduction, Multi-Hip	15x2
—	—	Pec Dec	12x2
—	—	Triceps Pressdown	12x2
—	—	Calf Raise, Standing	15x2
—	—	Prone Cobra	15x1
—	—	Treadmill	25 minutes, at 5-7 PRE

Weights — Week 2, Workout 2 (Mandatory)

—	—	Abdominal Crunch	15x2
—	—	Pulldown to Chest	12x2
—	—	Leg Press, Incline	12x2

Weights			
— —	Side Lateral Raise		12x2
— —	Adduction		15x3
— —	Bench Press, Incline Machine		10x2
— —	Triceps Pressdown		12x2
— —	Leg Extension		12x2
— —	Biceps Curl, Dumbbell		10x2
— —	Stairclimber	10 minutes, at 5-7 PRE	
— —	Treadmill	15 minutes, at 5-7 PRE	

Weights   Week 2, Workout 3 (Mandatory)

Weights			
— —	Pelvic Tilt		15x1
— —	Cross Crunch		15x1
— —	Lunge, Front		15x2
— —	Petersen Step-Up		15x2
— —	Military Press, Dumbbells		12x2
— —	Leg Curl, Prone		15x2
— —	One-Arm Row, Dumbbell		12x2
— —	Abduction, Multi-Hip Machine		15x2
— —	Pec Dec		12x2
— —	Triceps Pressdown		12x2
— —	Calf Raise, Standing		15x2
— —	Prone Cobra		15x1
— —	Treadmill	25 minutes, at 5-7 PRE	

Weights   Week 2, Workout 4 (Home, Optional)

Weights		
— —	Lunge, Reverse	8x4
— —	Push-Up	12x2
— —	Squat, Ballet	10x3
— —	Lunge, Stationary	10x3
— —	Chair Dips	10x3
— —	Lunge, Front	10x3

Comments: _____

_____

_____

Week Beginning:

_____

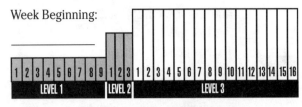

Level Two, Week 3

Frequency: Three days in the health club; one optional day at home

Rest Between Sets: 60 seconds

Rest Between Exercises: 45 seconds to two minutes

Tempo: For lower-body exercises, lower the weight in four seconds and lift in two seconds. For upper-body exercises, lower the weight in three seconds and lift in two seconds.

Comments: Are you starting to feel the *Lower Body Solution*? Don't worry, you won't always have sore legs, but oh those lunges can get you at first. This week it's the same ol' thing with a few extra sets.

Divide your week in a manner that fits your schedule. The workouts can be consecutive, or you can spread them out over the week. The optional home workout can fit in whenever it's convenient in your schedule, but not on the same day as a club workout.

The days that you don't work out should be considered "active rest" days. For me, that means I still try to stay very active. In the summer I love to water-ski; in the winter it's downhill skiing. In between, I love to ride my bike around the Napa Valley or go roller blading. The point is that you should try to stay (or become) active even on your days at rest. That may mean walking a little faster when you're working at your job or doing daily chores. It may be just parking farther from the store so you can powerwalk to your shopping.

A healthy lifestyle involves more than going to the gym every day. Try to make your rest "active"!

Weights   Week 3, Workout 1 (Mandatory)

Weights			
— —	Cross Crunch		15x1
— —	Lunge, Front		15x3
— —	Petersen Step-Up		15x3
— —	Military Press, Dumbbells		12x3
— —	Leg Curl, Prone		15x3
— —	One-Arm Row, Dumbbell		12x3
— —	Abduction, Multi-Hip Machine		15x3
— —	Pec Dec		12x3
— —	Triceps Pressdown		12x3
— —	Calf Raise, Standing		15x3
— —	Treadmill	15 minutes, at 6-8 PRE	
— —	Stairclimber	10 minutes, at 5-7 PRE	

Weights Week 3, Workout 2 (Mandatory)

__	__	Pelvic Tilt	15x1
__	__	Lunge, Front	15x3
__	__	Petersen Step-Up	15x3
__	__	Military Press, Dumbbells	12x3
__	__	Leg Curl, Prone	15x3
__	__	One-Arm Row, Dumbbell	12x3
__	__	Abduction, Multi-Hip Machine	15x3
__	__	Pec Dec	12x3
__	__	Triceps Pressdown	12x3
__	__	Calf Raise, Standing	15x3
__	__	Stairclimber	10 minutes, at 6-8 PRE
__	__	Treadmill	15 minutes, at 5-7 PRE

Weights Week 3, Workout 3 (Mandatory)

__	__	Cross Crunch	15x1
__	__	Lunge, Front	15x3
__	__	Petersen Step-Up	15x3
__	__	Military Press, Dumbbells	12x3
__	__	Leg Curl, Prone	15x3
__	__	One-Arm Row, Dumbbell	12x3
__	__	Abduction, Multi-Hip	15x3
__	__	Pec Dec	12x3
__	__	Triceps Pressdown	12x3
__	__	Calf Raise, Standing	15x3
__	__	Stairclimber	20 minutes, at 6-8 PRE

Weights Week 3, Workout 4 (Home, Optional)

__	__	Lunge, Reverse	8x4
__	__	Push-Up	12x2
__	__	Squat, Dumbbells	10x3
__	__	Lunge, Stationary	10x3
__	__	Chair Dip	10x3
__	__	Lunge, Front	10x3

Comments: _____

_____

_____

Level Three Workouts

For those who've worked their way up to this level and for those lucky enough to be able to begin at this point, let me welcome you along for a workout program like none you've ever done before.

Most importantly, let me welcome you to a program that will finally produce the results you've been waiting for.

This is the *Lower Body Solution*. As I've already said, it is designed to take the stubborn weight off your lower body, but it will also result in general weight loss. Like me, you may find your upper body shrinking at first, but don't worry, the lower body will follow next!

This is a four-month program. At the end of this program you will have noticeably changed your body. You will lose weight and you will gain muscle tone. Your thighs, hips, belly and buttocks will all shrink in size.

Maximum Flexibility

The program is designed with three mandatory days and two optional days in the health club and one optional day at home. With this flexibility you should be able to get through the four months to reap the rewards. Be sure to take your baseline measurements and bodyweight now, then check them every week or two to chart your progress (I know, you'll check them practically every day no matter what I say!)

Okay, on with the show.

Week Beginning:

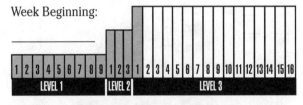

Level Three, Week 1

Frequency: Three mandatory days in the health club (can be consecutive); two optional health club days; one optional home day (in any particular order).

Rest Between Sets: 45 seconds

Rest Between Exercises: 45 seconds to two minutes

Tempo: For lower-body exercises, lower the weight in four seconds and lift in two seconds. For upper-body exercises, lower the weight in three seconds and lift in two seconds.

Comments: This program changes almost weekly. This first week starts you off easy. Think of an undulating curve. That's how the *Lower Body Solution* works to get the weight off. You'll go from easy to hard, to easy and back to hard.

You may notice some soreness. Warm baths and an anti-inflammatory such as aspirin will help. If you become so sore as to be nearly incapacitated, you need to cut down on the intensity of the exercise by reducing the resistance you work against, or in the case of the lunge, reducing the total number of repetitions. This program is designed to ease you into it. Don't try to jump ahead, or you'll really need that aspirin!

Take a few minutes to cross-reference the exercises in this routine with the descriptions in the Exercise

Index. Optional exercises are suggested if the prescribed movements cause pain or discomfort, or for other reasons cannot be performed. The descriptions in the Exercise Index offer some other options as well.

Weights	Week 1, Workout 1 (Mandatory)	Reps/Sets
__ __	Double Leg Lowering	15x1
__ __	Lunge, Stationary	15x2
__ __	One-Arm Row, Seated with Cable	12x2
__ __	Lunge, Reverse, with Cable	15x2
__ __	Close-Grip Pulldown, Parallel Grip	12x2
__ __	Squat, Smith Machine	15x2
__ __	Stationary Bicycle 25 minutes, at 5-7 PRE	

Weights	Week 1, Workout 2 (Mandatory)	
__ __	Side Bend, Dumbbell	15x1
__ __	Leg Press, Inclined	15x2
__ __	Bench Press, Incline Machine	12x2
__ __	Lunge Walk	15x2
__ __	Prone Triceps Extension	12x2
__ __	Leg Extension	15x2
__ __	Leg Press Calf Raise	15x2
__ __	Treadmill 25 minutes, at 5-7 PRE	

Weights	Week 1, Workout 3 (Mandatory)	
__ __	Double Leg Lowering	15x1
__ __	Lunge, Stationary	15x2
__ __	One-Arm Row, Seated, with Cable	12x2
__ __	Lunge, Reverse, with Cable	15x2
__ __	Close-Grip Pulldown, Parallel Grip	12x2
__ __	Squat, Smith Machine	15x2
__ __	Stationary Bicycle 25 minutes, at 5-7 PRE	

Weights	Week 1, Workout 4 (Optional)	
__ __	Side Bend, Dumbbell	15x1
__ __	Leg Press, Inclined	15x2
__ __	Bench Press, Incline Machine	12x2
__ __	Lunge Walk	15x2
__ __	Prone Triceps Extension	12x2
__ __	Leg Extension	15x2
__ __	Leg Press Calf Raise	15x2
__ __	Treadmill 25 minutes, at 5-7 PRE	

Weights	Week 1, Workout 5 (Optional)	
__ __	Double Leg Lowering	15x1
__ __	Lunge, Stationary	15x2
__ __	One-Arm Row, Seated, with Cable	12x2
__ __	Lunge, Reverse, with Cable	15x2
__ __	Close-Grip Pulldown, Parallel Grip	12x2
__ __	Squat, Smith Machine	15x2
__ __	Stationary Bicycle 25 minutes, at 5-7 PRE	

Weights	Week 1, Workout 6 (Optional Home or Health Club)	
__ __	Lunge, Reverse	15x4
__ __	Push-Up	12x2
__ __	Squat, Ballet	15x3
__ __	Lunge, Stationary	15x3
__ __	Chair Dip	12x3
__ __	Lunge, Front	15x3

*Perceived Rate of Exertion (for a full explanation, see Chapter 10)

Comments: _____

_____

_____

Week Beginning:

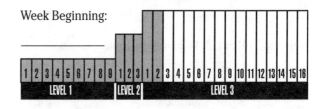

Level Three, Week 2

Frequency: Three mandatory days in the health club (can be consecutive); two optional health club days; one optional home day (in any particular order).

Rest Between Sets: 45 seconds

Rest Between Exercises: 45 seconds to two minutes

Tempo: For lower-body exercises, lower the weight in four seconds and lift in two seconds. For upper-body exercises, lower the weight in three seconds and lift in two seconds.

Comments: So how did you do last week? Three, four, five or did you actually manage to get in six workouts? If you did, I bet it wasn't as difficult as you suspected.

There's a lot more work this week, but that's what you're here for. The exercises are the same as last week, but you now have three sets on most of the major muscle groups. The routine is ordered so that your lactic acid levels stay normal, which means it won't "burn" when you're performing the routine, but you should be feeling some soreness the following days. Hang in there; you're going to get a break real soon.

From last week you should be familiar with the proper weights to use. The poundages may go up, or down, on some of your lifts this week. Make that third set count, every time. And remember, you can do anything for just one more set! Be sure to put effort into your weight training; you can't sleepwalk through these routines and expect results.Use your rest times to stop, think about the lift, rehearse it in your mind, then do it with some gusto!

If you haven't already, this would be a good time to write down your body measurements and weight. Weigh yourself at the beginning of each day, always at the same time, and always naked. Your bodyweight fluctuates too much during the day to give you an accurate idea of what is happening to your fat. And remember, muscle weighs more than fat so in the beginning you may not see a big change in your bodyweight. Instead, the initial changes may be in your measurements.

Weights	Week 2, Workout 1 (Mandatory)	
__ __	Double Leg Lowering	15x1
__ __	Lunge, Stationary	15x3
__ __	One-Arm Row, Seated, with Cable	12x3
__ __	Lunge, Reverse, with Cable	15x3
__ __	Close-Grip Pulldown, Parallel Grip	12x3
__ __	Squat, Smith Machine	15x3
__ __	Stairclimber	25 minutes, at 5-7 PRE

Wts	Week 2, Workout 2 (Mandatory)	
__ __	Side Bend, Dumbbell	15x1
__ __	Leg Press, Inclined	15x3
__ __	Bench Press, Incline Machine	12x3
__ __	Lunge Walk	15x3
__ __	Prone Triceps Extension	12x3
__ __	Leg Extension	15x3
__ __	Leg Press Calf Raise	15x3
__ __	Stationary Bike	25 minutes, at 5-7 PRE

Weights	Week 2, Workout 3 (Mandatory)	
__ __	Crunch Machine	20x1
__ __	Squat, Smith Machine	20x2
__ __	Close-Grip Pulldown, Parallel Grip	15x2
__ __	Lunge, Reverse, with Cable	20x2

__ __	One-Arm Row, Seated, with Cable	15x2
__ __	Lunge, Stationary	20x2
__ __	Treadmill	15 minutes, at 6-8 PRE
__ __	Stairclimber	25 minutes, at 5-7 PRE

Weights	Week 2, Workout 4 (Optional)	
__ __	Side Bend, Dumbbell	15x1
__ __	Leg Press, Inclined	15x3
__ __	Bench Press, Incline Machine	12x3
__ __	Lunge Walk	15x3
__ __	Prone Triceps Extension	12x3
__ __	Leg Extension	15x3
__ __	Leg Press Calf Raise	15x3
__ __	Stationary Bike	25 minutes, at 5-7 PRE

Weights	Week 2, Workout 5 (Optional)	
__ __	Double Leg Lowering	15x1
__ __	Lunge, Stationary	15x3
__ __	One-Arm Row, Seated, with Cable	12x3
__ __	Lunge, Reverse, with Cable	15x3
__ __	Close-Grip Pulldown, Parallel Grip	12x3
__ __	Squat, Smith Machine	15x3
__ __	Stairclimber	25 minutes, at 5-7 PRE

Weights	Week 2, Workout 6 (Optional Home or Health Club)	
__ __	Lunge, Reverse	15x4
__ __	Push-Up	12x2
__ __	Squat, Ballet	15x3
__ __	Lunge, Stationary	15x3
__ __	Chair Dip	12x3
__ __	Lunge, Front	15x3

Comments: _____

_____

_____

Week Beginning:

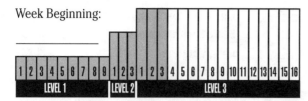

1	2	3	4	5	6	7	8	9	1	2	3	1	2	3	4	5	6	7	8	9	10	11	12	13	14	15	16

LEVEL 1   LEVEL 2   LEVEL 3

Level Three, Week 3

Frequency: Three mandatory workouts; three optional workouts

Rest Between Sets: 45 seconds

Rest Between Exercises: 45 seconds to two minutes

Tempo: For lower-body exercises, lower the weight in four seconds and lift in two seconds. For upper-body exercises, lower the weight in three seconds and lift in two seconds.

Comments: This is your last week of this workout phase. If you're getting tired, remember, you can do anything for one more week!

How many days a week are you managing to work out? If you've been averaging more than three then you deserve big congratulations! If you're still struggling with schedules, turn back to Chapter 7 and try working in more home workouts to get your frequency up.

If you've been managing four, five or even six days a week you are well on your way to turning your body into a fat-burning machine. Check out Chapter 15 and try to get your diet on the right track with your workouts. You may even want to use some of my fat-burning supplement suggestions. The *Lower Body Solution* is just starting to kick in, and this is indeed one of the most exciting things you've done for yourself in a long, long time.

Weights	Week 3, Workout 1 (Mandatory)	
__ __	Double Leg Lowering	15x1
__ __	Lunge, Stationary	15x3
__ __	One-Arm Row, Seated, with Cable	12x3
__ __	Lunge, Reverse, with Cable	15x3
__ __	Close-Grip Pulldown, Parallel Grip	12x3
__ __	Squat, Smith Machine	15x3
__ __	Treadmill 25 minutes, at 6-8 PRE	

Weights	Week 3, Workout 2 (Mandatory)	
__ __	Side Bend, Dumbbell	15x1
__ __	Leg Press, Inclined	15x3
__ __	Bench Press, Barbell	12x3
__ __	Lunge Walk	15x3
__ __	Prone Triceps Extension	12x3
__ __	Leg Extension	15x3
__ __	Leg Press Calf Raise	15x3
__ __	Stairclimber 25 minutes, at 6-8 PRE	

Weights	Week 3, Workout 3 (Mandatory)	
__ __	Crunch Machine	20x1
__ __	Squat, Smith Machine	20x2
__ __	Close-Grip Pulldown, Parallel Grip	15x2
__ __	Lunge, Reverse, with Cable	20x2
__ __	One-Arm Row, Seated, with Cable	15x2
__ __	Lunge, Stationary	20x2
__ __	Stairclimber 35 minutes, at 5-7 PRE	

Weights	Week 3, Workout 4 (Optional)	
__ __	Side Bend, Dumbbell	15x1
__ __	Leg Press, Inclined	15x3
__ __	Bench Press, Barbell	12x3
__ __	Lunge Walk	15x3
__ __	Prone Triceps Extension	12x3
__ __	Leg Extension	15x3
__ __	Leg Press Calf Raise	15x3
__ __	Stairclimber 25 minutes, at 6-8 PRE	

Weights	Week 3, Workout 5 (Optional)	
__ __	Double Leg Lowering	15x1
__ __	Lunge, Stationary	15x3
__ __	One-Arm Row, Seated, with Cable	12x3
__ __	Lunge, Reverse, with Cable	15x3
__ __	Close-Grip Pulldown, Parallel Grip	12x3
__ __	Squat, Smith Machine	15x3
__ __	Treadmill 25 minutes, at 6-8 PRE	

Weights	Week 3, Workout 6 (Home, Optional)	
__ __	Step-Up	15x3
__ __	Chair Dip	12x3
__ __	Lunge, Front	15x2
__ __	Push-Up	12x2
__ __	Lunge, Stationary	15x3
__ __	Pelvic Tilt	15x2
__ __	Abdominal Crunch	15x3

Comments: _____

_____

_____

1	2	3	4	5	6	7	8	9	1	2	3	1	2	3	4	5	6	7	8	9	10	11	12	13	14	15	16
LEVEL 1									**LEVEL 2**			**LEVEL 3**															

Level Three, Week 4

Frequency: Three mandatory days in the health club (can be consecutive), two optional health club days; one optional home day (in any particular order).

Rest Between Sets: 30 seconds

Rest Between Exercises: two to three minutes

Tempo: For lower-body exercises, lower the weight in four seconds and lift in two seconds. For upper-body exercises, lower the weight in three seconds and lift in two seconds.

Comments: Congratulations on completing the first three weeks of level three. You are now capable of performing many more exercises because you have strengthened the important core muscle groups that perform all the basic movements.

Week 4 begins a two-week interval program that will really help shock the fat off your lower body. If you've never performed this type of training before, get ready to sweat!

You'll also notice that for these two weeks you'll be performing more sets and lower reps. This modification is designed to match the intensity level of the interval training for optimal effectiveness. In other words, you are into this program with both feet and ready to turn into a fat-burning machine. Go girl!

Weights	Week 4, Workout 1 (Mandatory)	
— —	Cable Crunch	10x1
— —	Lunge, Stationary	10x3
— —	Military Press, Dumbbells	8x3
— —	Leg Press, Horizontal	10x3
— —	Leg Curl, Seated	10x3
— —	Triceps Pressdown	8x3
— —	Rowing Machine, Seated	8x3
— —	Calf Raise, Seated	10x3
— —	Prone Cobra	10x1
— —	Stationary Bike	5 minutes, at 5-7 PRE
		5 minutes, at 8-9 PRE
— —	Treadmill	5 minutes, at 5-7 PRE
		5 minutes, at 8-9 PRE
— —	Stairclimber	5 minutes, at 5-7 PRE

Weights	Week 4, Workout 2 (Mandatory)	
— —	Double Leg Lowering	10x1
— —	Petersen Step-Up	10x3
— —	Pec Dec	8x3
— —	Lunge Walk	10x3
— —	One-Arm Row, Dumbbell	8x3
— —	Upright Row, Dumbbells	8x3
— —	Hip Extension, Multi-Hip Machine	10x3
— —	Calf Raise, Standing	10x3
— —	Back Extension	10x1
— —	Treadmill	5 minutes, at 5-7 PRE
		5 minutes, at 8-9 PRE
		5 minutes, at 5-7 PRE
		5 minutes, at 8-9 PRE
		5 minutes, at 5-7 PRE

Weights	Week 4, Workout 3 (Mandatory)	
— —	Cable Crunch	10x1
— —	Lunge, Stationary	10x3
— —	Military Press, Dumbbells	8x3
— —	Leg Press, Horizontal	10x3
— —	Leg Curl, Seated	10x3
— —	Triceps Pressdown	8x3
— —	Rowing Machine, Seated	8x3
— —	Calf Raise, Seated	10x3
— —	Prone Cobra	10x1
— —	Stationary Bike	5 minutes, at 5-7 PRE
		5 minutes, at 8-9 PRE
— —	Treadmill	5 minutes, at 5-7 PRE
		5 minutes, at 8-9 PRE
— —	Stairclimber	5 minutes, at 5-7 PRE

Weights	Week 4, Workout 4 (Optional)	
— —	Double Leg Lowering	10x1
— —	Petersen Step-Up	10x3
— —	Pec Dec	8x3
— —	Lunge Walk	10x3
— —	One-Arm Row, Dumbbell	8x3
— —	Upright Row, Dumbbells	8x3
— —	Hip Extension, Multi-Hip Machine	10x3
— —	Calf Raise, Standing	10x3
— —	Back Extension	10x1
— —	Treadmill	5 minutes, at 5-7 PRE
		5 minutes, at 8-9 PRE
		5 minutes, at 5-7 PRE
		5 minutes, at 8-9 PRE
		5 minutes, at 5-7 PRE

Weights	Week 4, Workout Six (Optional, Home)	
— —	Lunge, Front	15x2
— —	Plié Position One	10x2
		5 seconds down, 2 up
— —	Plié Position Two	10x2
		5 seconds down, 2 up

—	—	Plié Position Three	10x2
		5 seconds down, 2 up	
—	—	Plié Position Four	10x2
		5 seconds down, 2 up	
—	—	Plié Position One	10x2
		5 seconds down, 2 up	
		Hamstring Stretch	
		Quadriceps Stretch	

Comments: _____

_____

_____

Week Beginning:

_____

Level Three, Week 5

Frequency: Three mandatory days in the health club (can be consecutive); two optional health club days; one optional home day (in any particular order).

Rest Between Sets: 30 seconds

Rest Between Exercises: two to three minutes

Tempo: For lower-body exercises, lower the weight in four seconds and lift in two seconds. For upper-body exercises, lower the weight in three seconds and lift in two seconds.

Comments: Didn't I tell you the interval training would make you sweat? Okay, one more week to go.

Are you feeling as though the weights are adding some bulk? No fear, the cardio workouts following your weight training make bulking up nearly impossible on this program. However, as you begin feeding new muscle fibers you become more aware of your muscles, and that often produces a "feeling" that they're getting larger. More toned, yes; larger, not likely.

Watch closely the rest between your sets. Only 30 seconds; count it off and get right back to the exercise. Okay, here you go for another cardio interval week.

Weights		Week 5, Workout 1 (Mandatory)	
—	—	Cable Crunch	10x1
—	—	Lunge, Stationary	10x4
—	—	Military Press, Dumbbells	8x4
—	—	Leg Press, Horizontal	10x4
—	—	Leg Curl, Seated	10x4
—	—	Triceps Pressdown	8x4
—	—	Rowing Machine, Seated	8x4
—	—	Calf Raise, Seated	10x4

—	—	Prone Cobra	10x1
—	—	Stationary Bike	5 minutes, at 5-7 PRE
			5 minutes, at 8-9 PRE
—	—	Treadmill	5 minutes, at 5-7 PRE
			5 minutes, at 8-9 PRE
—	—	Stairclimber	5 minutes, at 5-7 PRE
			5 minutes, at 6-8 PRE
			5 minutes, at 5-7 PRE

Weights		Week 5, Workout 2 (Mandatory)	
—	—	Cross Crunch	10x1
—	—	Petersen Step-Up	10x4
—	—	Pec Dec	8x4
—	—	Lunge Walk	10x4
—	—	One-Arm Row, Dumbbell	8x4
—	—	Upright Row, Dumbbells	8x4
—	—	Hip Extension, Multi-Hip Machine	10x4
—	—	Calf Raise, Standing	10x4
—	—	Back Extension	10x1
—	—	Stationary Bike	5 minutes, at 5-7 PRE
			5 minutes, at 8-9 PRE
			5 minutes, at 5-7 PRE
			5 minutes, at 8-9 PRE
			5 minutes, at 5-7 PRE

Weights		Week 5, Workout 3 (Mandatory)	
—	—	Cable Crunch	10x1
—	—	Lunge, Stationary	10x4
—	—	Military Press, Dumbbells	8x4
—	—	Leg Press, Horizontal	10x4
—	—	Leg Curl, Seated	10x4
—	—	Triceps Pressdown	8x4
—	—	Rowing Machine, Seated	8x4
—	—	Calf Raise, Seated	10x4
—	—	Prone Cobra	10x1
—	—	Stairclimber	5 minutes, at 5-7 PRE
			5 minutes, at 8-9 PRE
			5 minutes, at 5-7 PRE
			5 minutes, at 8-9 PRE
			5 minutes, at 5-7 PRE

Weights		Week 5, Workout 4 (Optional)	
—	—	Cross Crunch	10x1
—	—	Petersen Step-Up	10x4
—	—	Pec Dec	8x4
—	—	Lunge Walk	10x4
—	—	One-Arm Row, Dumbbell	8x4
—	—	Upright Row, Dumbbells	8x4
—	—	Hip Extension, Multi-Hip Machine	10x4
—	—	Calf Raise, Standing	10x4

		Back Extension	10x1
—	—	Stationary Bike	5 minutes, at 5-7 PRE 5 minutes, at 8-9 PRE
—	—	Treadmill	5 minutes, at 5-7 PRE 5 minutes, at 8-9 PRE
—	—	Stairclimber	5 minutes, at 5-7 PRE 5 minutes, at 6-8 PRE 5 minutes, at 5-7 PRE

Weights	Week 5, Workout 5 (Optional)	
— —	Cable Crunch	10x1
— —	Lunge, Stationary	10x4
— —	Military Press, Dumbbells	8x4
— —	Leg Press, Horizontal	10x4
— —	Leg Curl, Seated	10x4
— —	Triceps Pressdown	8x4
— —	Rowing Machine, Seated	8x4
— —	Calf Raise, Seated	10x4
— —	Prone Cobra	10x1
— —	Stairclimber	5 minutes, at 5-7 PRE 5 minutes, at 8-9 PRE 5 minutes, at 5-7 PRE 5 minutes, at 8-9 PRE 5 minutes, at 5-7 PRE

Weights	Week 5, Workout 6 (Optional, Home)	
— —	Lunge, Front	10x2
— —	Plié Position One	10x2 5 seconds down, 2 up
— —	Plié Position Two	10x2 5 seconds down, 2 up
— —	Plié Position Three	10x2 5 seconds down, 2 up
— —	Plié Position Four	10x2 5 seconds down, 2 up
— —	Plié Position One	10x2 5 seconds down, 2 up
	Hamstring Stretch	
	Quadriceps Stretch	

Comments: _____

_____

_____

Week Beginning:

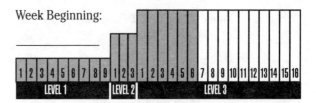

Level Three, Week 6

Frequency: Three mandatory days in the health club (can be consecutive); two optional health club days; one optional home day (in any particular order).

Rest Between Sets: 60 seconds

Rest Between Exercises: One to two minutes

Tempo: For lower-body exercises, lower the weight in four seconds and lift in two seconds. For upper-body exercises, lower the weight in three seconds and lift in two seconds.

Comments: Now that you've experienced high-intensity interval training, it's time to make a big switch and try a week of medium-intensity aerobics. The cardio is 10 minutes longer than your normal sessions, but the extra time really makes a difference by digging deep into your fat-burning system.

You'll also notice that you'll be performing more reps and fewer sets this week for the weight training exercises. This modification is designed to match the intensity level of the cardio training for optimal effectiveness. If you feel headache, nausea or dizziness from these ultra-high reps, increase the rest interval between sets. Gradually decrease this interval until your body has become accustomed to the intensity and can handle the shorter rest intervals.

Are you starting to see why this routine is different from other programs you've been on? Be sure to cross-reference the exercises in the Exercise Index to make certain you are performing them in the precise fashion prescribed. Double-check rest intervals and try to follow the workouts in the exact order prescribed.

Have you been taking measurements and checking your weight? You should definitely be seeing the positive results you've longed for, and the best is yet to come!

Weights	Week 6, Workout 1 (Mandatory)	
— —	Side Bend, Dumbbell	20x1
— —	Lunge Walk	20x2
— —	Bench Press, Incline Machine	15x2
— —	Leg Press, Inclined	20x2
— —	Prone Triceps Extension	15x2
— —	Leg Extension	20x2
— —	Leg Press Calf Raise	20x2
— —	Treadmill	35 minutes, at 5-7 PRE

Weights	Week 6, Workout 2 (Mandatory)	
— —	Crunch Machine	20x1
— —	Squat, Smith Machine	20x2
— —	Close-Grip Pulldown,	
	Parallel Grip	15x2
— —	Lunge, Reverse, with Cable	20x2
— —	One-Arm Row,	
	Seated, with Cable	15x2
— —	Lunge, Stationary	20x2
— —	Stairclimber	35 minutes, at 5-7 PRE

Weights	Week 6, Workout 3 (Mandatory)	
— —	Side Bend, Dumbbell	20x1
— —	Lunge Walk	20x2
— —	Bench Press, Incline Machine	15x2
— —	Leg Press, Inclined	20x2
— —	Prone Triceps Extension	15x2
— —	Leg Extension	20x2
— —	Leg Press Calf Raise	20x2
— —	Treadmill	35 minutes, at 5-7 PRE

Weights	Week 6, Workout 4 (Optional)	
— —	Crunch Machine	20x1
— —	Squat, Smith Machine	20x2
— —	Close-Grip Pulldown,	
	Parallel Grip	15x2
— —	Lunge, Reverse, with Cable	20x2
— —	One-Arm Row	
	Seated, with Cable	15x2
— —	Lunge, Stationary	20x2
— —	Stairclimber	35 minutes, at 5-7 PRE

Weights	Week 6, Workout 5 (Optional)	
— —	Side Bend, Dumbbell	20x1
— —	Lunge Walk	20x2
— —	Bench Press, Incline Machine	15x2
— —	Leg Press, Inclined	20x2
— —	Prone Triceps Extension	15x2
— —	Leg Extension	20x2
— —	Leg Press Calf Raise	20x2
— —	Treadmill	35 minutes, at 5-7 PRE

Weights	Week 6, Workout 6 (Optional, Home)	
— —	Lunge, Front and Side	8x4
— —	Lunge, Stationary	15x2
— —	Push-Up	8x3
— —	Chair Dip	10x3

— —	Rear Leg Kick	15x3
— —	Pelvic Tilt	15x2
— —	Abdominal Crunch	20x3
— —	Prone Cobra	20 seconds, twice

Comments: _____

_____

_____

Week Beginning:

_____

Level Three, Week 7

Frequency: Three mandatory days in the health club (can be consecutive); two optional health club days; one optional home day (in any particular order).

Rest Between Sets: 30 seconds

Rest Between Exercises: 45 seconds to two minutes

Tempo: For lower-body exercises, lower the weight in four seconds and lift in two seconds. For upper-body exercises, lower the weight in three seconds and lift in two seconds.

Comments: The next three weeks are similar to weeks 1 through 3, but you'll notice that the rest between sets has decreased from 45 to just 30 seconds, and the intensity of the cardio has increased from 5-7 PRE to 6-8. Don't worry, you're ready for it!

How many workouts are you managing each week? Are you keeping track of your workouts and the weights you are using? Be sure to use this book as a journal. When you flip back through the pages you can see how far you've come in what really is just a few short weeks.

Weights	Week 7, Workout 1 (Mandatory)	
— —	Side Bend, Dumbbell	15x1
— —	Lunge, Front	15x2
— —	Bench Press, Incline Machine	12x2
— —	Leg Press, Horizontal	15x2
— —	Abduction, Multi-Hip	15x2
— —	Triceps Pressdown	12x2
— —	Close-Grip Pulldown,	12x2
	Parallel Grip	
— —	Calf Raise, Seated	15x2
— —	Prone Cobra	15x1
— —	Stationary Bike	25 minutes, at 6-8 PRE

Weights	Week 7, Workout 2 (Mandatory)	
__ __	Straight-Arm Pulldown	15x1
__ __	Step-Up	15x2
__ __	Pec Dec	12x2
__ __	Deadlift, Dumbbell	15x2
__ __	Chin-Up Machine	12x2
__ __	(opt. Pulldown to Chest	12x2)*
__ __	Upright Row, Dumbbells	12x2
__ __	Adduction, Multi-Hip Machine	15x2
__ __	Calf Raise, Standing	15x2
__ __	Back Extension	15x1
__ __	Treadmill 25 minutes, at 6-8 PRE	

Weights	Week 7, Workout 3 (Mandatory)	
__ __	Side Bend, Dumbbell	15x1
__ __	Lunge	15x2
__ __	Bench Press, Incline Machine	12x2
__ __	Leg Press, Horizontal	15x2
__ __	Abduction, Multi-Hip Machine	15x2
__ __	Triceps Pressdown	12x2
__ __	Close-Grip Pulldown, Parallel Grip	12x2
__ __	Calf Raise, Seated	15x2
__ __	Prone Cobra	15x1
__ __	Stationary Bike 25 minutes, at 6-8 PRE	

Weights	Week 7, Workout 4 (Optional)	
__ __	Straight-Arm Pulldown	15x1
__ __	Step-Up	15x2
__ __	Pec Dec	12x2
__ __	Deadlift, Dumbbell	15x2
__ __	Chin-Up Machine	12x2
__ __	(opt. Close-Grip Pulldown	12x2)
__ __	Upright Row, Dumbbells	12x2
__ __	Adduction, Multi-Hip Machine	15x2
__ __	Calf Raise, Standing	15x2
__ __	Back Extension	15x1
__ __	Treadmill 25 minutes, at 6-8 PRE	

Weights	Week 7, Workout 5 (Optional)	
__ __	Side Bend, Dumbbell	15x1
__ __	Lunge, Front	15x2
__ __	Bench Press, Incline Machine	12x2
__ __	Leg Press, Horizontal	15x2
__ __	Abduction, Multi-Hip	15x2
__ __	Triceps Pressdown	12x2

	Close-Grip Pulldown, Parallel Grip	12x2
__ __	Calf Raise, Seated	15x2
__ __	Prone Cobra	15x1
__ __	Stationary Bike 25 minutes, at 6-8 PRE	

Weights	Week 7, Workout 6 (Optional, Home)	
__ __	Lunge, Front and Side	8x4
__ __	Lunge, Stationary	15x2
__ __	Push-Up	12x3
__ __	Chair Dip	12x3
__ __	Rear Leg Kick	15x3
__ __	Pelvic Tilt	15x2
__ __	Abdominal Crunch	20x3
__ __	Prone Cobra	15x2

*Optional Exercise, less difficult

Comments: _____

_____

_____

Week Beginning:

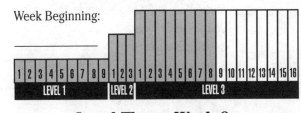

Level Three, Week 8

Frequency: Three mandatory days in the health club (can be consecutive); two optional health club days; one optional home day (in any particular order).

Rest Between Sets: 30 seconds

Rest Between Exercises: 45 seconds to two minutes

Tempo: For lower-body exercises, lower the weight in four seconds and lift in two seconds. For upper-body exercises, lower the weight in three seconds and lift in two seconds.

Comments: Last week you performed only two sets of the major weight training exercises. Break's over— you're back to three sets. Your rest between sets is only 30 seconds; stick to it!

Did you start a calendar to keep track of your workouts? If you did, then you can see we've been almost two months on the program so far. That means we are nearly one-third of the way through, and this is really where the fun begins.

Can you make a list of all the things that have changed in your body and in your life so far? Are you feeling more confident that the body of your dreams may finally be within your reach? It is; just stick with the program. It works.

Weights   Week 8, Workout 1 (Mandatory)

__	__	Side Bend, Dumbbell	15x1
__	__	Lunge, Reverse	15x3
__	__	Pec Dec	12x3
__	__	Leg Press, Horizontal	15x3
__	__	Abduction, Multi-Hip Machine	15x3
__	__	Triceps Pressdown	12x3
__	__	Close-Grip Pulldown, Parallel Grip	12x3
__	__	Calf Raise, Seated	15x3
__	__	Prone Cobra	15x1
__	__	Stairclimber 25 minutes, at 6-8 PRE	

Weights   Week 8, Workout 2 (Mandatory)

__	__	Straight-Arm Pulldown	15x1
__	__	Step-Up	15x3
__	__	Pec Dec	12x3
__	__	Lunge, Reverse, from Bench	15x3
__	__	Chin-Up Machine	12x3
__	__	(opt. Pulldown to Chest	12x3)
__	__	Biceps Curl, Dumbbells	12x3
__	__	Adduction, Multi-Hip Machine	15x3
__	__	Calf Raise, Standing	15x3
__	__	Back Extension	15x1
__	__	Stationary Bike 25 minutes, at 6-8 PRE	

Weights   Week 8, Workout 3 (Mandatory)

__	__	Side Bend, Dumbbell	15x1
__	__	Lunge, Reverse	15x3
__	__	Chair Dip	12x3
__	__	Leg Press, Horizontal	15x3
__	__	Abduction, Multi-Hip Machine	15x3
__	__	Triceps Pressdown	12x3
__	__	Close-Grip Pulldown, Parallel Grip	12x3
__	__	Calf Raise, Seated	15x3
__	__	Prone Cobra	15x1
__	__	Stairclimber 25 minutes, at 6-8 PRE	

Weights   Week 8, Workout 4 (Optional)

__	__	Straight-Arm Pulldown	15x1
__	__	Step-Up	15x3
__	__	Pec Dec	12x3
__	__	Lunge, Reverse, from Bench	15x3
__	__	Chin-Up Machine	12x3
__	__	(opt. Pulldown to Chest	12x3)
__	__	Biceps Curl, Dumbbells	12x3

__	__	Adduction, Multi-Hip Machine	15x3
__	__	Calf Raise, Standing	15x3
__	__	Back Extension	15x1
__	__	Stationary Bike 25 minutes, at 6-8 PRE	

Weights   Week 8, Workout 5 (Optional)

__	__	Side Bend, Dumbbell	15x1
__	__	Lunge, Reverse	15x3
__	__	Bench Press, Incline Machine	12x3
__	__	Leg Press, Horizontal	15x3
__	__	Abduction, Multi-Hip Machine	15x3
__	__	Triceps Pressdown	12x3
__	__	Close-Grip Pulldown, Parallel Grip	12x3
__	__	Calf Raise, Seated	15x3
__	__	Prone Cobra	15x1
__	__	Stairclimber 25 minutes, at 6-8 PRE	

Weights   Week 8, Workout 6 (Optional, Home)

__	__	Lunge, Reverse	8x4
__	__	Lunge, Stationary	15x2
__	__	Push-Up	12x3
__	__	Chair Dip	12x3
__	__	Rear Leg Kick	15x3
__	__	Pelvic Tilt	15x2
__	__	Abdominal Crunch	20x3
__	__	Prone Cobra	15x2

Comments: _____

_____

_____

Week Beginning: _____

1 2 3 4 5 6 7 8 9	1 2 3	1 2 3 4 5 6 7 8 9 10 11 12 13 14 15 16
LEVEL 1	LEVEL 2	LEVEL 3

Level Three, Week 9

Rest Between Sets: 30 seconds

Rest Between Exercises: 45 seconds to two minutes

Tempo: For lower-body exercises, lower the weight in four seconds and lift in two seconds. For upper-body exercises, lower the weight in three seconds and lift in two seconds.

Comments: This is the last week of this three-week phase. Next week will be another hard-core aerobic workout to accelerate fat-burning. Remember, you can do anything for just one more week!

Be sure to continue to cross-reference the Exercise Index in the back of the book. Even if you've been performing many of these exercises for a while now, it always helps to double-check your form. You may also be ready for some of the optional variations that are given in the back of the book.

Weights	Week 9, Workout 1 (Mandatory)	
___ ___	Side Bend, Dumbbell	15x1
___ ___	Lunge, Stationary	15x3
___ ___	Pec Dec	12x3
___ ___	Leg Press, Horizontal	15x3
___ ___	Abduction, Multi-Hip Machine	15x3
___ ___	Triceps Extension and Press	12x3
___ ___	Close-Grip Pulldown, Parallel Grip	12x3
___ ___	Calf Raise, Seated	15x3
___ ___	Prone Cobra	15x1
___ ___	Stairclimber	25 minutes, at 6-8 PRE

Weights	Week 9, Workout 2 (Mandatory)	
___ ___	Cross Crunch	15x1
___ ___	Step-Up	15x3
___ ___	Pec Dec	12x3
___ ___	Deadlift, Dumbbell	15x3
___ ___	Chin-Up Machine	12x3
___ ___	(opt. Close-Grip Pulldown, Parallel Grip	12x3)
___ ___	Upright Row, Dumbbells	12x3
___ ___	Adduction, Multi-Hip Machine	15x3
___ ___	Calf Raise, Standing	15x3
___ ___	Back Extension	15x1
___ ___	Stationary Bike	25 minutes, at 6-8 PRE

Weights	Week 9, Workout 3 (Mandatory)	
___ ___	Side Bend, Dumbbell	15x1
___ ___	Lunge, Stationary	15x3
___ ___	Pec Dec	12x3
___ ___	Leg Press, Horizontal	15x3
___ ___	Abduction, Multi-Hip Machine	15x3
___ ___	Triceps Extension and Press	12x3
___ ___	Close-Grip Pulldown, Parallel Grip	12x3
___ ___	Calf Raise, Seated	15x3
___ ___	Prone Cobra	15x1
___ ___	Stairclimber	25 minutes, at 6-8 PRE

Weights	Week 9, Workout 4 (Optional)	
___ ___	Cross Crunch	15x1
___ ___	Step-Up	15x3
___ ___	Pec Dec	12x3
___ ___	Deadlift, Dumbbell	15x3
___ ___	Chin-Up Machine	12x3
___ ___	(opt. Pulldown to Chest	12x3)
___ ___	Upright Row, Dumbbells	12x3
___ ___	Adduction, Multi-Hip Machine	15x3
___ ___	Calf Raise, Standing	15x3
___ ___	Back Extension	15x1
___ ___	Stationary Bike	25 minutes, at 6-8 PRE

Weights	Week 9, Workout 5 (Optional)	
___ ___	Side Bend, Dumbbell	15x1
___ ___	Lunge, Stationary	15x3
___ ___	Pec Dec	12x3
___ ___	Leg Press, Horizontal	15x3
___ ___	Abduction, Multi-Hip Machine	15x3
___ ___	Triceps Extension and Press	12x3
___ ___	Close-Grip Pulldown, Parallel Grip	12x3
___ ___	Calf Raise, Seated	15x3
___ ___	Prone Cobra	15x1
___ ___	Stairclimber	25 minutes, at 6-8 PRE

Weights	Week 9, Workout 6 (Optional, Home)	
___ ___	Double Leg Lowering	15x2
___ ___	Lunge, Stationary	15x2
___ ___	Push-Up	12x3
___ ___	Lunge, Reverse	15x2
___ ___	Chair Dip	12x3
___ ___	Step-Up	15x2
___ ___	Squat, Ballet	15x2
___ ___	Pelvic Tilt	15x2
___ ___	Abdominal Crunch	25x2
___ ___	Horse Stance	3x1 (Hold for 10 seconds)

Comments: _____

_____

_____

Week Beginning:

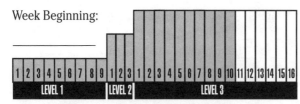

_____

| 1 | 2 | 3 | 4 | 5 | 6 | 7 | 8 | 9 | 1 | 2 | 3 | 1 | 2 | 3 | 4 | 5 | 6 | 7 | 8 | 9 | 10 | 11 | 12 | 13 | 14 | 15 | 16 |

| LEVEL 1 | LEVEL 2 | LEVEL 3 |

Level Three, Week 10

Rest Between Sets: 60 seconds
Rest Between Exercises: One to two minutes
Tempo: For lower-body exercises, lower the weight in four seconds and lift in two seconds. For upper-body exercises, lower the weight in three seconds and lift in two seconds.

Comments: Here you go again-another hard-core aerobic phase. Notice that you are performing fewer sets in the weight training workout; this is to help keep your workout time to about an hour.

This routine utilizes high repetitions, so you may start feeling a bit of a "burn" from the weight training phases. Notice also that your rest between sets has doubled to one minute. Count it out, and use that time to psyche yourself up for the next set.

You're in the heart of the *Lower Body Solution* workout. Your body is geared up for maximum fat-burning. Try to keep your calories in check and eat as well as you can. How about a few of those supplements to enhance the effects of the *Lower Body Solution*? Remember, the only way to achieve dramatic weight loss is through a combination of the right exercise program (this is it!) and lowered caloric consumption.

Weights	Week 10, Workout 1 (Mandatory)	
__ __	Double Leg Lowering	20x1
__ __	Squat, Smith Machine	20x2
__ __	Close-Grip Pulldown, Parallel Grip	15x2
__ __	Lunge, Reverse, with Cable	20x2
__ __	One-Arm Row, Seated, with Cable	15x2
__ __	Lunge, Stationary	20x2
__ __	Stationary Bike 35 minutes, at 5-7 PRE	

Weights	Week 10, Workout 2 (Mandatory)	
__ __	Side Bend, Dumbbell	20x1
__ __	Lunge Walk	20x2
__ __	Bench Press, Incline Machine	15x2
__ __	Leg Press, Inclined	20x2
__ __	Biceps Curl, Dumbbells	15x2
__ __	Leg Extension	20x2
__ __	Leg Press Calf Raise	20x2
__ __	Treadmill 35 minutes, at 5-7 PRE	

Weights	Week 10, Workout 3 (Mandatory)	
__ __	Double Leg Lowering	20x1
__ __	Squat, Smith Machine	20x2
__ __	Close-Grip Pulldown, Parallel Grip	15x2
__ __	Lunge, Reverse, with Cable	20x2
__ __	One-Arm Row, Seated, with Cable	15x2
__ __	Lunge, Stationary	20x2
__ __	Stationary Bike 35 minutes, at 5-7 PRE	

Weights	Week 10, Workout 4 (Optional)	
__ __	Side Bend, Dumbbell	20x1
__ __	Lunge Walk	20x2
__ __	Bench Press, Incline Machine	15x2
__ __	Leg Press, Inclined	20x2
__ __	Biceps Curl, Dumbbells	15x2
__ __	Leg Extension	20x2
__ __	Leg Press Calf Raise	20x2
__ __	Treadmill 35 minutes, at 5-7 PRE	

Weights	Week 10, Workout 5 (Optional)	
__ __	Double Leg Lowering	20x1
__ __	Squat, Smith Machine	20x2
__ __	Close-Grip Pulldown, Parallel Grip	15x2
__ __	Lunge, Reverse, with Cable	20x2
__ __	One-Arm Row, Seated, with Cable	15x2
__ __	Lunge, Stationary	20x2
__ __	Stationary Bike 35 minutes, at 5-7 PRE	

Weights	Week 10, Workout 6 (Optional, Home)	
__ __	Double Leg Lowering	15x2
__ __	Lunge, Stationary	15x2
__ __	Push-Up	12x3
__ __	Lunge, Reverse	15x2
__ __	Chair Dip	12x3
__ __	Step-Up	10x2
__ __	Squat, Dumbbells	10x2
__ __	Pelvic Tilt	15x2
__ __	Abdominal Crunch	25x2
__ __	Horse Stance 3x1(Hold for 10 seconds)	

Comments: _____

_____

_____

Week Beginning:

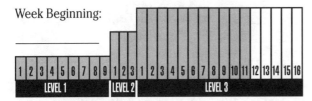

	1	2	3	4	5	6	7	8	9	1	2	3	1	2	3	4	5	6	7	8	9	10	11	12	13	14	15	16
LEVEL 1										LEVEL 2			LEVEL 3

Level Three, Week 11

Rest Between Sets: 30 seconds
Rest Between Exercises: 45 seconds to two minutes
Tempo: For lower-body exercises, lower the weight in four seconds and lift in two seconds. For upper-body exercises, lower the weight in three seconds and lift in two seconds.

Comments: Wow! After last week, you deserve a little break, and this is it. This three-week workout phase is similar to Weeks 1-3 and 7-9, with the first week containing only two sets of the major weight training exercises.

Are you hanging in there with the rest of us? How about frequency? Remember that truly stubborn fat on the hips and thighs is not only the last to go, but it also requires five- and six-day-a-week workouts to burn it off. Chapter 7 has several home workouts you can use for those weeks when you simply can't make it to the gym.

And how about those days off? Are you trying to employ the "active rest" principle and keep your body moving even on your days off? If the weather permits, walks are a wonderful way to get some exercise and meet some of your neighbors. If you can get out in the fresh air once a day, you've already got a leg up on fitness that many people seem to miss. How about just moving through your day with a little more bounce in your step? Every extra bit of energy you put out means more calories burned.

Weights — Week 11, Workout 1 (mandatory)

Weights	Exercise	Sets/Reps
__ __	Cross Crunch	15x1
__ __	Petersen Step-Up	15x2
__ __	Pec Dec	12x2
__ __	Lunge Walk	15x2
__ __	One-Arm Row, Dumbbell	12x2
__ __	Upright Row, Dumbbells	12x2
__ __	Hip Extension, Multi-Hip Machine	15x2
__ __	Calf Raise, Standing	15x2
__ __	Back Extension	15x1
__ __	Stairclimber	25 minutes, at 6-8 PRE

Weights — Week 11, Workout 2 (Mandatory)

Weights	Exercise	Sets/Reps
__ __	Cable Crunch	15x1
__ __	Lunge, Stationary	15x2
__ __	Military Press, Dumbbells	12x2
__ __	Lunge, Bench on Smith Machine	15x3
__ __	Leg Curl, Seated	15x2
__ __	Triceps Extension and Press	12x2
__ __	Rowing Machine, Seated	12x2
__ __	Calf Raise, Seated	15x2
__ __	Prone Cobra	15x1
__ __	Stationary Bike	25 minutes, at 6-8 PRE

Weights — Week 11, Workout 3 (Mandatory)

Weights	Exercise	Sets/Reps
__ __	Cross Crunch	15x1
__ __	Squat, Ballet	15x2
__ __	Pec Dec	12x2
__ __	Lunge Walk	15x2
__ __	One-Arm Row, Dumbbell	12x2
__ __	Upright Row, Dumbbells	12x2
__ __	Hip Extension, Multi-Hip Machine	15x2
__ __	Calf Raise, Standing	15x2
__ __	Back Extension	15x1
__ __	Stairclimber	25 minutes, at 6-8 PRE

Weights — Week 11, Workout 4 (Optional)

Weights	Exercise	Sets/Reps
__ __	Cable Crunch	15x1
__ __	Lunge, Stationary	15x2
__ __	Military Press, Dumbbells	12x2
__ __	Lunge, Bench, on Smith Machine	15x3
__ __	Leg Curl, Seated	15x2
__ __	Triceps Extension and Press	12x2
__ __	Rowing Machine, Seated	12x2
__ __	Calf Raise, Seated	15x2
__ __	Prone Cobra	15x1
__ __	Stationary Bike	25 minutes, at 6-8 PRE

Weights — Week 11, Workout 5 (Optional)

Weights	Exercise	Sets/Reps
__ __	Cross Crunch	15x1
__ __	Petersen Step-Up	15x2
__ __	Pec Dec	12x2
__ __	Lunge Walk	15x2
__ __	One-Arm Row, Dumbbell	12x2
__ __	Upright Row, Dumbbells	12x2
__ __	Hip Extension, Multi-Hip Machine	15x2
__ __	Calf Raise, Standing	15x2
__ __	Back Extension	15x1
__ __	Stairclimber	25 minutes, at 6-8 PRE

Weights — Week 11, Workout 6 (Optional, Home)

Weights	Exercise	Sets/Reps
__ __	Lunge, Front and Side	8x4
__ __	Lunge, Stationary	15x2
__ __	Push-Up	12x3

___	___	Chair Dip	12x3
___	___	Rear Leg Kick	15x3
___	___	Pelvic Tilt	15x2
___	___	Abdominal Crunch	20x3
___	___	Prone Cobra	15x2

Comments: _____

_____

_____

Week Beginning:

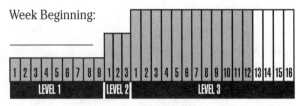

Level Three, Week 12

Rest Between Sets: 30 seconds

Rest Between Exercises: 45 seconds to two minutes

Tempo: For lower-body exercises, lower the weight in four seconds and lift in two seconds. For upper-body exercises, lower the weight in three seconds and lift in two seconds.

Comments: Time to check your progress. I bet you're feeling as though you could triple your cardio times, and you probably could! You are now more savvy about weight training exercises than most of the members at your health club. Way to go!

Contained in each of these routines are special exercises to improve the small postural muscles of the back. Are you practicing better posture with more ease now? You should be feeling at your physical best, and if you want to add a bit more cardio to your workouts now is the time to do it.

Extended cardio times will burn additional fat. If you are feeling up for it, you may want to extend two or three of your cardio sessions to last up to 65 minutes at this point. When and if you do, you are going to start to see pounds melting off you at an amazing rate. This is the point I upped my cardio considerably, and I was managing a two- to three-pound loss for the next three weeks.

It's meltdown time!

Weights	Week 12, Workout 1 (Mandatory)	
___ ___	Cross Crunch	15x1
___ ___	Petersen Step-Up	15x3
___ ___	Pec Dec	12x3
___ ___	Lunge Walk	15x3
___ ___	One-Arm Row, Dumbbell	12x3
___ ___	Upright Row, Dumbbells	12x3

___	___	Hip Extension, Multi-Hip Machine	15x3
___	___	Calf Raise, Standing	15x3
___	___	Back Extension	15x1
___	___	Treadmill	25 minutes, at 6-8 PRE

Weights	Week 12, Workout 2 (Mandatory)	
___ ___	Cable Crunch	15x1
___ ___	Lunge, Stationary	15x3
___ ___	Military Press, Dumbbells	12x3
___ ___	Leg Press, Horizontal	15x3
___ ___	Leg Curl, Seated	15x3
___ ___	Triceps Pressdown	12x3
___ ___	Rowing Machine, Seated	12x3
___ ___	Calf Raise, Seated	15x3
___ ___	Prone Cobra	15x1
___ ___	Stairclimber	25 minutes, at 6-8 PRE

Weights	Week 12, Workout 3 (Mandatory)	
___ ___	Cross Crunch	15x1
___ ___	Squat, Ballet	15x3
___ ___	Pec Dec	12x3
___ ___	Lunge Walk	15x3
___ ___	One-Arm Row, Dumbbell	12x3
___ ___	Upright Row, Dumbbells	12x3
___ ___	Hip Extension, Multi-Hip Machine	15x3
___ ___	Calf Raise, Standing	15x3
___ ___	Back Extension	15x1
___ ___	Treadmill	25 minutes, at 6-8 PRE

Weights	Week 12, Workout 4 (Optional)	
___ ___	Cable Crunch	15x1
___ ___	Lunge, Stationary	15x3
___ ___	Military Press, Dumbbells	12x3
___ ___	Leg Press, Horizontal	15x3
___ ___	Leg Curl, Seated	15x3
___ ___	Triceps Pressdown	12x3
___ ___	Rowing Machine, Seated	12x3
___ ___	Calf Raise, Seated	15x3
___ ___	Prone Cobra	15x1
___ ___	Stairclimber	25 minutes, at 6-8 PRE

Weights	Week 12, Workout 5 (Optional)	
___ ___	Cross Crunch	15x1
___ ___	Petersen Step-Up	15x3
___ ___	Pec Dec	12x3
___ ___	Lunge Walk	15x3
___ ___	One-Arm Row, Dumbbell	12x3

—	—	Upright Row, Dumbbells	12x3
—	—	Hip Extension, Multi-Hip Machine	15x3
—	—	Calf Raise, Standing	15x3
—	—	Back Extension	15x1
—	—	Treadmill	25 minutes, at 6-8 PRE

Weights **Week 12, Workout 6 (Optional, Home)**

—	—	Lunge, Front and Side	8x4
—	—	Lunge, Stationary	15x2
—	—	Push-Up	12x3
—	—	Chair Dip	12x3
—	—	Rear Leg Kick	15x3
—	—	Pelvic Tilt	15x2
—	—	Abdominal Crunch	20x3
—	—	Prone Cobra	15x2

Comments: _____

_____

_____

Week Beginning:

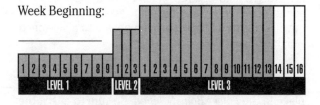

Level Three, Week 13

Rest Between Sets: 30 seconds

Rest Between Exercises: 45 seconds to two minutes

Tempo: For lower-body exercises, lower the weight in four seconds and lift in two seconds. For upper-body exercises, lower the weight in three seconds and lift in two seconds.

Comments: One week to go, then you're set to enjoy a week of the toughest aerobic training workouts in the program!

You're moving at a fast pace through your workouts and you can bet that every muscle fiber in your body is set at its highest fat-burning level. Try to keep the frequency up on your workouts—that is still key to your ultimate success.

Don't let your concentration wander in the gym. Make certain that from the moment you step through the door you are focused on the task that lies ahead. While doing your cardio, reread some of the success stories. Go back and check your own notes and congratulate yourself on the progress you've made thus far. Keep it up; it's working!

Weights **Week 13, Workout 1 (Mandatory)**

—	—	Russian Twist	15x1
—	—	Lunge, Bench, on Smith Machine	15x3
—	—	Dips, Machine	12x3
—	—	(opt. Bench Press, Incline Machine	12x3)
—	—	Lunge Walk	15x3
—	—	Upright Row, Dumbbells	12x3
—	—	Biceps Curl, Dumbbells	12x3
—	—	Hip Extension, Multi-Hip Machine	15x3
—	—	Calf Raise, Standing	15x3
—	—	Back Extension	15x1
—	—	Stationary Bike	25 minutes, at 6-8 PRE

Weights **Week 13, Workout 2 (Mandatory)**

—	—	Rugby Sit-Up	15x1
—	—	Lunge, Stationary	15x3
—	—	Military Press, Dumbbells	12x3
—	—	Leg Press, Horizontal	15x3
—	—	Leg Curl, Seated	15x3
—	—	Triceps Extension and Press	12x3
—	—	Rowing Machine, Seated	12x3
—	—	Calf Raise, Seated	15x3
—	—	Prone Cobra	15x1
—	—	Treadmill	25 minutes, at 6-8 PRE

Weights **Week 13, Workout 3 (Mandatory)**

—	—	Russian Twist	15x1
—	—	Lunge, Bench, on Smith Machine	15x3
—	—	Dips, Machine	12x3
—	—	(opt. Bench Press, Incline Machine	12x3)
—	—	Lunge Walk	15x3
—	—	Upright Row, Dumbbells	12x3
—	—	Biceps Curl, Dumbbells	12x3
—	—	Hip Extension, Multi-Hip Machine	15x3
—	—	Calf Raise, Standing	15x3
—	—	Back Extension	15x1
—	—	Stationary Bike	25 minutes, at 6-8 PRE

Weights	Week 13, Workout 4 (Optional)	
__ __	Rugby Sit-Up	15x1
__ __	Lunge, Stationary	15x3
__ __	Military Press, Dumbbells	12x3
__ __	Leg Press, Horizontal	15x3
__ __	Leg Curl, Seated	15x3
__ __	Triceps Extension and Press	12x3
__ __	Rowing Machine, Seated	12x3
__ __	Calf Raise, Seated	15x3
__ __	Prone Cobra	15x1
__ __	Treadmill	25 minutes, at 6-8 PRE

Weights	Week 13, Workout 5 (Optional)	
__ __	Russian Twist	15x1
__ __	Lunge, Reverse, from Bench	15x3
__ __	Dips, Machine	12x3
__ __	(opt. Bench Press, Incline Machine	12x3)
__ __	Lunge Walk	15x3
__ __	Upright Row, Dumbbells	12x3
__ __	Biceps Curl, Dumbbells	12x3
__ __	Hip Extension, Multi-Hip Machine	15x3
__ __	Calf Raise, Standing	15x3
__ __	Back Extension	15x1
__ __	Stationary Bike	25 minutes, at 6-8 PRE

Weights	Week 13, Workout 6 (Optional, Home)	
__ __	Double Leg Lowering	15x2
__ __	Lunge, Stationary	15x2
__ __	Push-Up	12x3
__ __	Lunge, Reverse	15x2
__ __	Chair Dip	12x3
__ __	Step-Up	15x2
__ __	Squat, Ballet	15x2
__ __	Pelvic Tilt	15x2
__ __	Abdominal Crunch	25x2
__ __	Horse Stance	3x1
		(Hold for 10 seconds)

Comments: _____

_____

_____

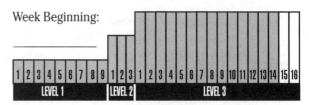

Week Beginning:

_____

Level Three, Week 14

Rest Between Sets: 60 seconds

Rest Between Exercises: One to two minutes

Tempo: For lower-body exercises, lower the weight in four seconds and lift in two seconds. For upper-body exercises, lower the weight in three seconds and lift in two seconds.

Comments: You're back to hard-core cardio, 40 minutes a day of fat-burning fun! You're also nearing the end of the 16-week program, and I bet you can hardly remember those first few workouts. But try to, and then start counting the improvements you've seen in the past months.

You may also want to flip forward and look at a few of the exercises in Chapter 16. These advanced movements can begin to replace some of the other exercises for more variety, if you feel ready for them. You may also have found a few workout phases that are your favorites by now. After week 16, you may want to spend some extra time on your favorite phases. You have at this point moved from a novice to a seasoned weight trainer.

This routine once again uses some new moves, exercises that aren't generally included in most bodybuilding routines, but exercises that have a definite place in the *Lower Body Solution*. Be sure to check the descriptions in the back of the book in order to perform these exercises properly.

Weights	Week 14, Workout 1 (Mandatory)	
__ __	Wood Chop, Seated	20x1
__ __	Leg Press, Inclined	20x2
__ __	Bench Press, Barbell	15x2
__ __	Lunge Walk	20x2
__ __	Prone Triceps Extension	15x2
__ __	Leg Extension	20x2
__ __	Leg Press Calf Raise	20x2
__ __	Stairclimber	40 minutes, at 5-7 PRE

Weights	Week 14, Workout 2 (Mandatory)	
__ __	Rugby Sit-Up	20x1
__ __	Lunge, Stationary	20x2
__ __	One-Arm Row, Seated, with Cable	15x2
__ __	Lunge, Reverse, with Cable	20x2
__ __	Close-Grip Pulldown, Parallel Grip	15x2

		Squat, Hack or Smith Machine	20x2
—	—	Stationary Bike 40 minutes, at 5-7 PRE	

Weights **Week 14, Workout 3 (Mandatory)**

—	—	Russian Twist	20x1
—	—	Leg Press, Inclined	20x2
—	—	Bench Press, Barbell	15x2
—	—	Lunge Walk	20x2
—	—	Prone Triceps Extension	15x2
—	—	Leg Extension	20x2
—	—	Leg Press Calf Raise	20x2
—	—	Stairclimber 40 minutes, at 5-7 PRE	

Weights **Week 14, Workout 4 (Optional)**

—	—	Rugby Sit-Up	20x1
—	—	Lunge, Stationary	20x2
—	—	One-Arm Row, Seated, with Cable	15x2
—	—	Lunge, Reverse, with Cable	20x2
—	—	Close-Grip Pulldown, Parallel Grip	15x2
—	—	Squat, Smith Machine	20x2
—	—	Stationary Bike 40 minutes, at 5-7 PRE	

Weights **Week 14, Workout 5 (Optional)**

—	—	Russian Twist	20x1
—	—	Leg Press, Inclined	20x2
—	—	Bench Press, Barbell	15x2
—	—	Lunge Walk	20x2
—	—	Prone Triceps Extension	15x2
—	—	Leg Extension	20x2
—	—	Leg Press Calf Raise	20x2
—	—	Stairclimber 40 minutes, at 5-7 PRE	

Weights **Week 14, Workout 6 (Optional, Home)**

—	—	Lunge, Front and Side	8x4
—	—	Lunge, Stationary	15x2
—	—	Push-Up	8x3
—	—	Chair Dip	12x3
—	—	Rear Leg Kick	15x3
—	—	Pelvic Tilt	15x2
—	—	Abdominal Crunch	20x3
—	—	Prone Cobra	15x2

Comments: _____

_____

_____

Week Beginning:

_____

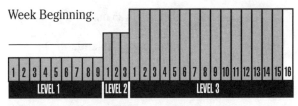

Level Three, Week 15

Rest Between Sets: 30 seconds
Rest Between Exercises: 45 seconds to two minutes
Tempo: For lower-body exercises, lower the weight in four seconds and lift in two seconds. For upper-body exercises, lower the weight in three seconds and lift in two seconds.

Comments: You're almost to the finish line. Are you planning a one- or two-week vacation when you're finished? Oh, did I forget that part? You don't have to start from week 1 immediately—as a matter of fact, a vacation from your workout is not only in order, I demand it!

As you've learned, your body responds better to a workout that is constantly changing. You've also learned that rest is as important to your workout as effort. When you complete week 16, take one or two weeks off the program, and when you restart at week 1 your body is going to be anxious and eager to jump back in with renewed energy and results!

Weights **Week 15, Workout 1 (Mandatory)**

—	—	Cross Crunch	15x1
—	—	Lunge, Gorsha	15x3
—	—	Pec Dec	12x3
—	—	Deadlift, Dumbbell	15x3
—	—	Chin-Up Machine (opt. Close-Grip Pulldown, Parallel Grip)	12x3
—	—	Upright Row, Dumbbells	12x3
—	—	Adduction, Multi-Hip Machine	15x3
—	—	Calf Raise, Standing	15x3
—	—	Back Extension	15x1
—	—	Treadmill 25 minutes, at 6-8 PRE	

Weights **Week 15, Workout 2 (Mandatory)**

—	—	Side Bend, Dumbbell	15x1
—	—	Lunge, Reverse	15x3
—	—	Bench Press, Barbell	12x3
—	—	Leg Press, Horizontal	15x3
—	—	Abduction, Multi-Hip Machine	15x3
—	—	Triceps Pressdown	12x3
—	—	Close-Grip Pulldown, Parallel Grip	12x3
—	—	Calf Raise, Seated	15x3
—	—	Prone Cobra	15x1

___	___	Stairclimber	25 minutes, at 6-8 PRE

Weights		Week 15, Workout 3 (Mandatory)	
___	___	Cross Crunch	15x1
___	___	Lunge, Gorsha	15x3
___	___	Pec Dec	12x3
___	___	Deadlift, Dumbbell	15x3
___	___	Chin-Up Machine	12x3
___	___	(opt. Close-Grip Pulldown, Parallel Grip	12x3)
___	___	Upright Row, Dumbbells	12x3
___	___	Adduction, Multi-Hip Machine	15x3
___	___	Calf Raise, Standing	15x3
___	___	Back Extension	15x1
___	___	Treadmill	25 minutes, at 6-8 PRE

Weights		Week 15, Workout 4 (Optional)	
___	___	Side Bend, Dumbbell	15x1
___	___	Lunge, Reverse	15x3
___	___	Bench Press, Barbell	12x3
___	___	Leg Press, Horizontal	15x3
___	___	Abduction, Multi-Hip Machine	15x3
___	___	Triceps Pressdown	12x3
___	___	Close-Grip Pulldown, Parallel Grip	12x3
___	___	Calf Raise, Seated	15x3
___	___	Prone Cobra	15x1
___	___	Stairclimber	25 minutes, at 6-8 PRE

Weights		Week 15, Workout 5 (Optional)	
___	___	Cross Crunch	15x1
___	___	Lunge, Gorsha	15x3
___	___	Pec Dec	12x3
___	___	Deadlift, Dumbbell	15x3
___	___	Chin-Up Machine	12x3
___	___	(opt. Close-Grip Pulldown, Parallel Grip	12x3)
___	___	Upright Row, Dumbbells	12x3
___	___	Adduction, Multi-Hip Machine	15x3
___	___	Calf Raise, Standing	15x3
___	___	Back Extension	15x1
___	___	Treadmill	25 minutes, at 6-8 PRE

Weights		Week 15, Workout 6 (Optional, Home)	
___	___	Lunge, Front and Side	8x4
___	___	Lunge, Stationary	15x2
___	___	Push-Up	12x3
___	___	Chair Dip	12x3
___	___	Rear Leg Kick	15x3
___	___	Pelvic Tilt	15x2
___	___	Abdominal Crunch	20x3
___	___	Prone Cobra	15x2

Comments: ______________________________

____

____

Week Beginning:

____

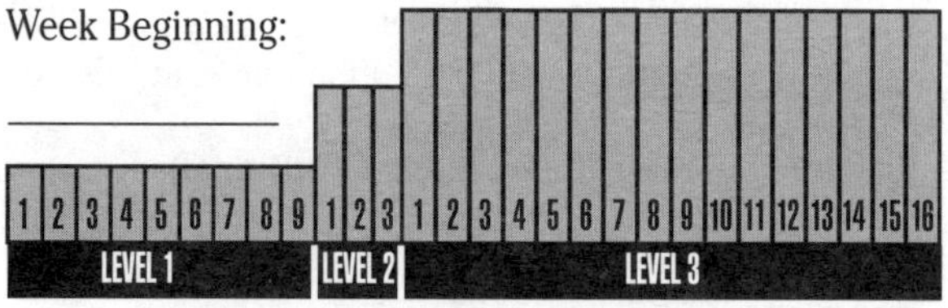

Level Three, Week 16

Rest Between Sets: 30 seconds

Rest Between Exercises: 45 seconds to two minutes

Tempo: For lower-body exercises, lower the weight in four seconds and lift in two seconds. For upper-body exercises, lower the weight in three seconds and lift in two seconds.

Comments: Congratulations! You've made it through the program!

How much weight have you lost? How many inches? How much stronger are you now??? If you've graduated through the levels, or if you were already in good shape and ready to tackle a brand new way of training for women only, you deserve a big high five and a pat on the back for completing the program.

Be certain to take your measurements, and if possible get an "after" photo. I'd love to see it.

Sixteen weeks is a long time, and I bet many of you didn't think you'd make it all the way through. In retrospect, it wasn't really that hard. One of the toughest things is making that first decision to do something about the shape you're in. That decision made, the rest is just follow through.

You can do anything for just one more week, so get back in the club and finish the program off with some enthusiasm. Then take a week or two off and buy a new outfit to go along with that new figure. When you resume your workouts, start to take all the knowledge you've gained about weight training, cardio and your own body, and use it to begin to fine-tune this program to give you the body you've always wanted. And remember, you're in this for the long haul. Getting older really can be about getting better.

Weights		Week 16, Workout 1 (Mandatory)	
___	___	Crunch Machine	15x1
___	___	Step-Up	15x3

Weights				

		Dip, Machine	12x3
—	—	(opt. Bench Press, Incline Machine	12x3)
—	—	Deadlift, Dumbbell	15x3
—	—	Chin-Up Machine	12x3
—	—	(opt. Pulldown to Chest	12x3)
—	—	Upright Row, Dumbbells	12x3
—	—	Adduction, Multi-Hip Machine	15x3
—	—	Calf Raise, Standing	15x3
—	—	Back Extension	15x1
—	—	Stationary Bike 25 minutes, at 6-8 PRE	

Weights   Week 16, Workout 2 (Mandatory)

		Wood Chop, Seated	15x1
—	—	Lunge, Side	15x3
—	—	Pec Dec	12x3
—	—	Lunge, Reverse from Bench	15x3
—	—	Abduction, Multi-Hip	15x3
—	—	Triceps Extension and Press	12x3
—	—	Close-Grip Pulldown, Parallel Grip	12x3
—	—	Calf Raise, Seated	15x3
—	—	Prone Cobra	15x1
—	—	Treadmill 25 minutes, at 6-8 PRE	

Weights   Week 16, Workout 3 (Mandatory)

		Crunch Machine	15x1
—	—	Step-Up	15x3
—	—	Dip, Machine	12x3
—	—	(opt. Bench Press, Incline Machine 12x3)	
—	—	Deadlift, Dumbbell	15x3
—	—	Chin-Up Machine	12x3
—	—	(opt. Close-Grip Pulldown, Parallel Grip)	
—	—	Upright Row, Dumbbells	12x3
—	—	Adduction, Multi-Hip Machine	15x3
—	—	Calf Raise, Standing	15x3
—	—	Back Extension	15x1
—	—	Stationary Bike 25 minutes, at 6-8 PRE	

Weights   Week 16, Workout 4 (Optional)

		Wood Chop, Seated	15x1
—	—	Lunge, Side	15x3
—	—	Pec Dec	12x3
—	—	Lunge, Reverse from Bench	15x3
—	—	Abduction, Multi-Hip Machine	15x3
—	—	Triceps Extension and Press	12x3
—	—	Close-Grip Pulldown, Parallel Grip	12x3
—	—	Calf Raise, Seated	15x3
—	—	Prone Cobra	15x1
—	—	Treadmill 25 minutes, at 6-8 PRE	

Weights   Week 16, Workout 5 (Optional)

		Crunch Machine	15x1
—	—	Step-Up	15x3
—	—	Dip, Machine	12x3
—	—	(opt. Bench Press, Incline Machine 12x3)	
—	—	Deadlift, Dumbbell	15x3
—	—	Chin-Up Machine	12x3
—	—	(opt. Pulldown to Chest	12x3)
—	—	Upright Row, Dumbbells	12x3
—	—	Adduction, Multi-Hip Machine	15x3
—	—	Calf Raise, Standing	15x3
—	—	Back Extension	15x1
—	—	Stationary Bike 25 minutes, at 6-8 PRE	

Weights   Week 16, Workout 6 (Optional, Home)

		Double Leg Lowering	15x2
—	—	Lunge, Stationary	15x2
—	—	Push-Up	12x3
—	—	Lunge, Reverse	15x2
—	—	Chair Dip	12x3
—	—	Step-Up	15x2
—	—	Squat, Dumbbells	15x2
—	—	Pelvic Tilt	15x2
—	—	Abdominal Crunch	25x2
—	—	Horse Stance	3x1

(Hold for 10 seconds)

Lower Body Stretch

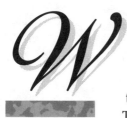omen live busy lives. The last thing we need is a stringent "you must be here at this time" workout regimen. That's why the *Lower Body Solution* offers you so many options to work out at home, to work out on consecutive days, to workout whenever and wherever you can.

Stretching is as important to your overall fitness as weight training and aerobics. It is excellent to stretch when your muscles are warm immediately following a workout, but that may add minutes to your workout time that you cannot afford. Therefore, this stretching program is designed to be done at your leisure. Personally, I enjoy stretching late in the evening, usually while watching the late news. It takes a little more time because I need to do a short warm-up before stretching, but its effects are almost as soothing as a hot tub when I'm done.

The benefits of stretching go beyond simply increasing flexibility. Stretching can make you feel more relaxed by reducing muscle tension. It can also prevent muscle strains, promote circulation, and prevent and even cure certain types of back pain. If that's not enough, how about just the fact that stretching feels good and only takes a few minutes a day! I know that stretching is not essential to burning fat, but it is an essential component of every weight training routine.

Stretching elongates a muscle. Weight training contracts a muscle. By following your *Lower Body Solution* workouts with stretching you eliminate that tight, bulked-up feeling you get from high-frequency lower body training. Your lower body stretching will help make your muscles become lithe and limber.

Although stretching is one of the safest types of exercise, there are a few conditions where you shouldn't stretch. Unless a physician or other competent medical provider says otherwise, you shouldn't stretch the muscles around a bone that's been recently fractured, or an area that has been recently sprained or strained—especially the muscles of the back or neck. Of course, if you have a question about the safety aspects of a specific stretch or stretching in general, you should consult your physician.

If you are not stretching immediately after your workout, you will need to perform a warm-up prior to stretching. I prefer to do five to ten minutes of low-intensity aerobic activity, such as a slow set of pliés followed by a set of stationary lunges or some light running in place to get my heart rate up. During the summer months I go outside on the back porch and do a few minutes of jump rope—that really helps me to break a sweat fast! Sit-ups are also good to help heat up your body temperature.

You should stretch in loose, comfortable clothing and without jewelry. A nonskid, firm mat is ideal for stretching, and the area you're stretching in should be quiet so you can concentrate. Finally, although stretching can be performed anywhere and anytime, it's probably not a good idea to stretch immediately after eating.

Over the years several theories have surfaced about the best ways to stretch. Unfortunately, some of these—such as holding your breath—were proposed by "greater-consciousness" types who were better suited to tell us how to stretch our minds than our muscles. Others, such as *Stretching* (Random House), the classic book on stretching by Bob Anderson, and Michael J. Alter's *Sport Stretch* (Human Kinetics), present good, solid guidelines to follow. The routine presented here is for the lower body; if you would like to add some upper body stretches I suggest you contact those references.

Here are a few guidelines that pertain to all stretching:
- Stretch slowly, moving smoothly into each stretch.
- Breathe normally as you stretch, but emphasize exhaling as you ease deeply into a stretch.
- Do not force a joint to the point that you feel pain, and do not extend a joint beyond its normal range of motion. Feel the stretch but don't make it torture.
- Hold each stretch for about 15 seconds.
- Ease out of every stretch smoothly and slowly.

As in the *Lower Body Solution* workout, variety is the key. You should periodically change the order of the stretches you perform. This is a basic routine for your lower body and you should add some upper body stretches to make it complete. In addition to changing your stretches periodically, you should also vary the orientation of your stretches. Every small adjustment in a stretch, even varying your arm position on a leg stretch, will hit different fibers in the muscle.

To get you started on a stretching program, here are nine stretches that work all the major muscles of the lower body.

Calf Stretch

Many women have tight calves because they spend so much time in high heels, tightness that can also irritate the sciatica nerve. This is an excellent exercise to help resolve both problems.

Stand about two feet away from a wall, facing it. Place your hands on the wall, or on your right knee as shown, arms straight and hips back. Move your left foot about two feet behind your right, trying to transfer the majority of your bodyweight to the ball of your left foot.

Begin the stretch by pressing your left heel to the floor and pushing your hips forward so that your torso is in line with your back leg. Do not allow the back foot to roll inward (pronate) as this places

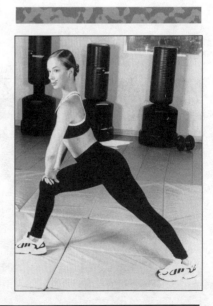

harmful stress on the Achilles tendon. Now increase the intensity of the stretch by contracting your left buttock, hold, then return to the start. Repeat for the other leg.

Contracting the buttocks, a technique popularized by strength coach Charles Poliquin, increases the value of the movement by stretching some of the connective tissues that often restrict flexibility.

Glute Stretch

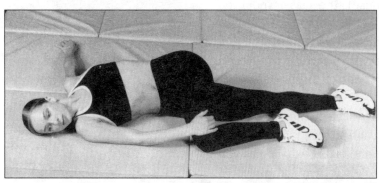

The glutes (buttocks) are worked hard in the *Lower Body Solution*, and this is a great movement to help you recover from intense workouts. It also stretches the lower back.

Lie on your back and flex your left leg so that the upper leg is perpendicular to the floor. Place your right hand on the outside of your left knee and extend your left arm out to the side, in line with your shoulders. This is the start position.

Perform the stretch by pulling the left leg over your right, using your right hand for leverage. As you pull, allow the left hip to come up also, but do not stretch so that you have to force the stretch or so far that your left shoulder lifts off the floor. Hold, return to the start, and repeat for the other side.

Another variation of the stretch that some individuals prefer is to look at your extended arm during the full stretch position. Do whichever technique you find most comfortable.

Some trainers recommend that you leave the hips on the floor throughout the entire stretch. This variation tends to excessively arch and twist the spine, effects that may cause or aggravate back pain.

Hamstring Stretch

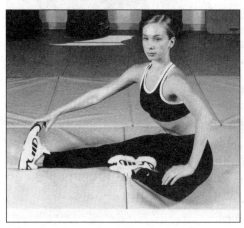

Because so many of us spend most of the day sitting on our hamstrings, this area tends to become very tight. Because tight hamstrings are often associated with lower back pain, it's wise to include at least one hamstring stretch in your workout.

The hamstrings consist of three muscles that extend from the back of the hips to the top of the calves. Because it's such a long muscle group, the best stretches for this area are performed with the leg straight.

Sit down on the floor, place your right foot out in front of you and pull in your left leg so that your left foot touches the inside of your right thigh. Place your right hand on the ball of your right foot, and your right hand on your left knee. Without

Lower Body Solution

rounding your back, lean forward as far as comfortable, hold, and then return to the start. Repeat for the other leg.

To more effectively stretch each of the three muscles of the hamstrings, rotate your extended leg inward and outward, keeping the leg straight as you do so. Thus, you could perform one repetition with your foot pointed straight up, one rep with your leg rotated inward, and one rep with your leg rotated outward.

If you find that your hamstrings are especially tight and it's difficult to maintain proper back posture, hook a towel over your arch and grasp the ends with both hands. If you hook the towel over the ball of your foot you can also really stretch the calves. To stretch the upper calf (gastrocnemius) keep the leg straight; to stretch the lower calf (soleus) bend your knee slightly.

Hip Flexor Stretch

This is probably the most underrated exercise for preventing and resolving back pain. It stretches the hip flexors, muscles on the front of the hip that help lift the leg and pull the trunk forward. When tight, the hip flexors rotate the pelvis forward, creating an excessive arch in the lower back that may cause pain and increase the risk of degenerative disorders of the spine. One way to determine if you have tight hip flexors is to lie face up with your legs straight. If you find this position uncomfortable, then you need this stretch.

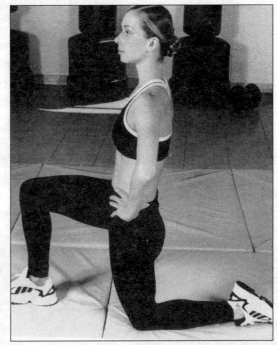

Kneel on your left knee, placing your right foot in front, in a split position, and put your hands on your hips. Your legs should be spread far enough apart so you feel a light stretch on the front of your right hip and upper leg. Keep your head level and look straight ahead. This is the start position.

Perform the stretch by rotating your pelvis down and forward, hold, then return to the start. To increase the range of motion of the stretch, and also to slightly stretch the upper abs, place your hands behind your head and lean back slightly, lifting your chest up and keeping your head in line with your torso. If this modification causes pain, then of course don't do it and stick with the standard version of this stretch.

Lower Back Stretch I (not shown)

Here's an easy stretch on the lower back and buttocks that feels great! Simply lie on your back, grasp the back of your right knee, and pull it to your chest so that your kneecap is in line with your armpit. (Do not perform this exercise by grasping the front of the knee as this can place harmful stress on the knee ligaments.) Hold and then return to the start. Also, for those who've had disc problems and found this exercise uncomfortable, often the discomfort can be resolved by placing a small towel, the diameter of your fist, under your lower back. This will prevent the discs of the lower back from irritating the nerves. Of course, you should always check with your doctor before performing any stretching routine designed to resolve back pain.

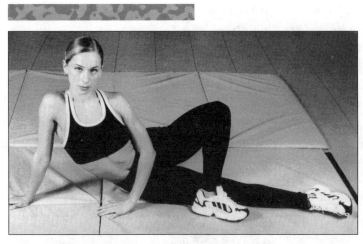

Oblique Stretch

This is a great stretch for the side abdominal muscles and the outside of the hip. If you look in a mirror and find that you have one hip higher than the other, this could indicate that these muscles are tight.

Lie on your right side and lift up your torso so that your shoulders are level, using your right arm for support. Place your left arm in front of you at your waist. Now bend your left leg and cross it over your right, positioning it alongside the knee. Finally, rotate the right leg so that the entire length of the right side of the foot is in contact with the floor. From this start position, simply push your right side down with your arms until you feel the stretch. Hold, then repeat for the other side.

To increase the stretch on the hip, perform the exercise with your extended leg resting on a low step.

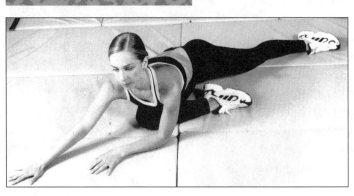

Piriformis Stretch

The piriformis is a hip muscle that rotates the hips and, when tight, is often found to be associated with sciatica. The piriformis can be a difficult muscle to stretch, but I have found this exercise to be excellent.

Kneel upright on the floor and bend your right leg in front of you, resting the knee on the floor. Extend your left leg behind you, and turn your upper body so that you are facing forward. Stay upright, using your arms to help. This is the start position.

Perform the exercise by leaning forward, keeping a slight arch in your back as you do so. As you lean forward, extend your arms in front of you for stability. Hold when you feel a comfortable stretch in your hips, then return to the start. Repeat for the other side.

Lower Back Stretch II

In addition to stretching the lower back throughout its entire length, this stretch also relaxes the muscles on the back of the neck. Because you're not lying on your back during this lower-back stretch, those with tight hip flexors may prefer this movement over the previous lower-back stretch.

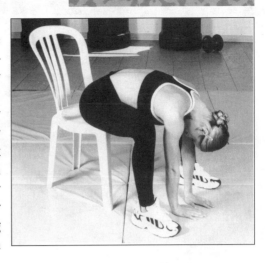

Sit on the edge of a chair, feet flat on the floor. Begin by placing your hands on your legs, and then dropping your head forward until you feel a comfortable stretch on the back of your neck. Increase the stretch by placing your elbows on your knees and allowing your back to round. Now place your hands on the floor, between your feet and in line with your heels, and allow your back to round; your head should hang freely. If possible, place your palms on the floor. Hold, then slowly return to the start, using your arms to assist you.

At no time during this exercise should you allow your back or neck to twist. And as stated earlier, you should always check with your doctor before performing any stretching routine designed to resolve back pain.

Quadriceps Stretch

Although this exercise doesn't require any special equipment, those with poor balance should perform it near a wall so they can place one hand on the wall to improve their stability.

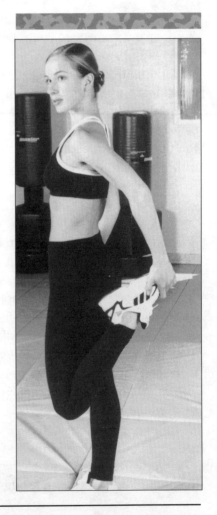

With your left hand, grasp the top of your left ankle and pull your foot towards your rear end as far as comfortable. In this position your upper thigh should be perpendicular to the floor, your chest should be up, and you should be looking straight ahead. Hold the stretch, keeping the lower leg aligned with the upper leg (there is a tendency to pull the lower leg away from the body, which could strain ligaments), then slowly return to the start. Repeat for the other leg.

To also stretch the shins, hold the toes rather than the ankle (as shown at right).

CHAPTER FIFTEEN

Effective Eating

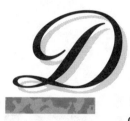iet is a dirty word. I prefer "effective eating." It has a nice sound. It also reminds us that what we eat has a direct affect on how we look.

Too many women are controlled by their food cravings and sweet tooth. When you think about food, rather than think about the satisfying taste, think about what's in it for you. That piece of chocolate cake can taste great, but a salmon filet pan-seared with a dab of butter and delicate spice can taste just as delicious and also provide you with high quality protein, artery-protecting cholesterol and other vitamins and nutrients. When you look at food, ask yourself "What can it do for me?"

This is a book about exercise and body mechanics. It is also a book about fighting fat and therefore must address the subject of diet. But, unlike the *Lower Body Solution* approach to exercise, there is not a single sure-fire approach to dieting for weight loss that will work for all women. There are many great diet programs out there, and I suggest that until you find a program that works you should continue to explore them all, even the kookiest ones.

The Food Dilemma
While struggling with my own weight, I confess to having at one time fallen for the biggest line of

hype the diet industry has ever produced: "Lose weight without dieting!" The product was Met-Rx, which at the time promised a "scientifically engineered food" that would spare the muscle and waste the fat.

Prices back then for this product were much higher, and I invested my first $150 and began using Met-Rx exactly as directed. So did my training partner at the time, Jackie. Using the program and working out according to the directions, we both gained weight, and quite a bit of it as I recall. When we stopped using Met-Rx, we both lost weight. So much for products that sell themselves with such hype.

Try Something New
I don't pretend to be an expert on dieting, but I will tell you what I have learned and what I recommend. The most important thing to do is keep an open mind and give almost everything a try. My esthetician had great results with a diet based on blood types. Another friend had immense success with Suzanne Somers' "eat all you want" diet. A client of mine enjoyed weight loss and renewed energy on the low-carbohydrate, high-fat Atkins diet.

I've tried grazing, that is, eating numerous small meals a day. I got fatter. I tried zero fat and then low fat. I still gained weight. I tried high carbohydrates and then I really gained weight. In the end, I went back to how I had eaten most of my life: lean meats and lots of vegetables. I had never been a big bread and pasta person (until I met my husband), and now I've gone back to eating the way I ate when I was slim. For my husband, the high carbohydrates are not a problem. They may not be a problem for you. They are for me.

Today my diet is low-fat (25 percent), medium protein (35 percent) and low carbohydrates (40 percent). I eat dinner out at least once a week and have learned to eat healthily. I consume as few empty calories as possible, such as alcoholic drinks and large desserts, although I almost always order dessert (but eat half of it or less).

Meal Replacement Drinks

I like these—a lot. I highly recommend meal replacement drinks, but not the ones designed for men and muscle building. I also have nothing against Slim Fast—it's better than pigging out on foods outside your diet plan and is usually available at any major grocery store. However, the meal replacements I recommend are significantly better than any available at the grocery store.

In my opinion you cannot use a better meal replacement than Slim Again's Weight Loss Shake by U.S. Nutriceuticals (1-877-292-6614). Right off the bat, I *love* the name of the product—nearly all of us have been slim at some point in our lives. I believe one of the simplest approaches to weight loss is to go back to eating the way you ate when you were slim.

However, my excitement about the Slim Again Weight Loss Shake goes far beyond the name. It is low in fat and low in high glycemic sugars. It is made with high quality soy protein, which I believe is beneficial to women of all ages, especially middle-age women. In addition to calcium and other vital vitamins and minerals, the shakes are loaded with the best ingredients known to promote weight loss. This includes CitriMax, an herbal ingredient that helps curb appetite, and ChromeMate which improves carbohydrate metabolism.

Slim Again's Weight Loss Shake also contains Calcium Pyruvate, one of the newest breakthroughs in weight loss. Studies have shown that dieters who use pyruvate lose more weight and keep it off longer. Slim Again's product takes things a step further by adding Pepti-Lean, a special micro-peptide blend of ingredients that controls fat metabolism. The clinical research on these ingredients is promising (nine percent body fat reduction in three months) and I believe the combination of ingredients in this shake is about the closest we've come to finding a dietary supplement that melts fat as well, if not better, than exercise.

When I'm actively trying to lose weight, I drink two of these a day. The success stories in Chapter Two told of a few of my clients' successes with the shakes and I could share with you many more. In my experience, they work.

New Breakthroughs

Exercise is definitely your first line of defense against fat. But right behind it is diet. While we're still a long way from discovering a pill to achieve healthy weight loss, new scientific breakthroughs have produced products that can make weight loss easier.

In addition to Slim Again's Weight Loss Shake there are two other exceptional products produced by the same company (U.S. Nutriceuticals 1-877-292-6614.) One of these is the Slim Again Diet Bar, which contains many of the same ingredients as the shake. As a matter of fact, I often eat a bar in lieu of a shake. Even when weight loss is not my prime objective, I eat these bars because I like their taste and they are loaded with fat-burning ingredients like CitriMax, Chrome-Mate and Pepti-Lean.

The other essential weight loss supplement in

Slim Again's product line is Pyru-Lean which contains pyruvate, Pepti-Lean and chromium. I first began using Pyruvex, a pyruvate supplement from SportPharma (1-800-292-6536) nearly a year ago. I found it to be the most effective fat-burning supplement I'd come across, until discovering Slim Again's Pyru-Lean. I use three capsules of the Pyru-Lean instead of six of the Pyruvex. Pyru-Lean's additional fat burners enhance the effectiveness of pyruvate.

Supplements for Success

In addition to the Slim Again products there are several other supplements I swear by. If I'm in a weight loss phase I take two L-Carnitine capsules (SportPharma 1-800-292-6536) before my workouts. During my workouts I drink Cutting Force, a fat-burning drink from American Body Building (1-800-627-0627). This drink also contains L-Carnitine and I use it even when I'm not actively dieting.

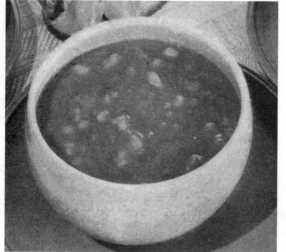

To round out my supplement arsenal I use a fiber drink. I believe that one of the key elements missing from the American diet is fiber—both soluble and insoluble. Studies have shown that insoluble fiber can attach itself to the "bad" cholesterol in the body and literally flush it out of the system. These findings have led some nutritionists to theorize that people in certain European countries can routinely eat a high-fat diet yet not suffer the high cholesterol and incidence of heart disease that we have in America.

The fiber drink I use is called Bios Life 2 (1-707-253-7227, ask for Phil) and I drink about three or four of these a week.

Laura's Cabbage Soup

Years ago I tried the Cabbage Soup diet and lost more than ten pounds in a week. Three weeks later, I'd managed to remain five pounds lighter. I know other people who simply hate the taste of the soup and swear they can't lose a single pound on it. Oh well, as I said, diets are an individual matter.

For me, seeing the scale drop by several pounds in a week is a great motivator. That's when I pull out my old Cabbage Soup recipe. I can usually tolerate two or three days of eating nothing but Cabbage Soup, my morning nonfat latte, mineral water, a Slim Again shake and bar, and one fiber drink, and—viola!—the pounds drop away! By day four I have one more bowl of soup and then resume my normal eating habits. For me, this little Cabbage Soup ritual always jump-starts my enthusiasm to put some extra effort into my workouts and extra care into my eating habits— both of which pay off in feeling healthier, more vital, energetic and slim!

My Cabbage Soup Concoction consists of six cups of water, two packs of Lipton Onion Soup mix, one very large onion, one bunch of celery, one medium bell pepper and two heads of cabbage. Dice all the vegetables; combine with soup mix and water. Bring it to a boil and simmer for about 45 minutes, then add salt and pepper to taste. I usually put the whole pot in the refrigerator and microwave small bowls whenever I'm hungry.

Women and Food

Women have a unique relationship with food, as evidenced by the startling prevalence of eating disorders among the female, but not the male, population. Eating disorders can be successfully treated, and thankfully, there are more resources for women to go to than ever before. Two resources on the subject I found particularly enlightening are books *The Obsession* and *The Hungry Self* by Kim Chernin, a Berkeley, California, counselor for women with eating disorders. In these books you'll find fascinating theories on how the way a woman relates to food mirrors the way she feels about herself. You'll also read about how frustrating it is for a woman to try to diet on a man's terms and deny herself foods that are so basic to her nature. If you have or suspect you have an eating disorder, I advise reading these books.

When You Eat

In addition to what you eat, *when* you eat affects the way you gain weight. Fasting two hours before bedtime helps most people cut calories. It is also an easy way to enhance your body's growth hormone production.

Growth hormone is produced primarily during sleep. Sugary carbohydrates before bedtime can interfere with sleep patterns and diminish its production. Growth hormone helps increase metabolism so that you burn fat more effectively. It is also responsible for a healthy fat-to-muscle ratio.

The Dieting Dilemma

No matter what I say, a certain percentage of you are going to practically starve yourself to get thin. I know you've heard this before, but starvation diets don't work. They backfire.

When women lose weight on diets that are extremely low in calories, their bodies go into a negative nitrogen balance, a condition that causes the body to break down muscle tissue for fuel. Losing just a pound of muscle through this process can result in as much as a 50-calorie reduction in calories burned per day.

Another problem that occurs with very-low-calorie diets is that the thyroid gland produces less of the biochemical triiodothyronine. Triiodothyronine helps regulate body temperature, which is one of the factors that determines your metabolism. The most accurate way to determine thyroid function is a blood test, but a more practical way is to check your morning body temperature. If your waking temperature is below 98 degrees, that could be an indication your thyroid may not be functioning normally and your metabolism is slowing down. (An extremely low morning body temperature may also be indicative of other health problems, so a visit to a doctor would be a wise decision.)

After the Diet

If you decide to use a reduced-calorie diet to lose weight, you need to wean yourself back to regular eating to avoid rebound weight gain. Depending upon how severe the diet was and how long you were on it, it may take up to three months of careful diet management to resume normal eating habits and to return thyroid levels to normal.

Gradually increasing your calories is one way to get back on track, but the best way to ensure that a rapid fat gain doesn't occur to use a rotation diet that varies calorie intake daily. For example, if you've followed a 700-calories-per-day diet for several weeks, you could wean yourself by alternating 900-, 1,200-, and 1,500-calories-per-day diets for several weeks before going back to a regular diet of 1,800 calories a day.

The Diet Basics

Everyone looks for the one best way to lose weight. Unfortunately, there is no single way that works for everyone. Every individual reacts differently to diets, and finding the right diet is often a trial-and-error process. Whether you choose the Pritikin Diet, the Zone, Cabbage Soup or the Rice Diet, there are certain general guidelines that, if followed, will help ensure the success of your diet.

■ Don't Use Starvation Diets

Many women develop problems with dieting because their calorie intake is too low, and because of this, their bodies seek (and find!) ways to protect their fat stores. Consulting with a nutritionist about the minimum number of calories you need to consume will help you avoid the Yo-Yo Syndrome.

■ Exercise More

The bottom line of weight loss is that you need to expend more calories than you consume. The best way to burn more calories is to exercise more. Whether it's through weight training (which also raises your metabolism by increasing muscle mass), aerobic exercise or physical games or activities, the point is to simply exercise more. A good guideline for weight loss is to increase whatever form of exercise you are currently performing by one third.

■ Eat Only When You're Hungry

Appetite is triggered by the brain, but we often eat out of habit without any real hunger cravings. We eat lunch at noon because everybody eats lunch at noon. We eat three meals a day because we've been told that's the way it is. We eat popcorn and candy and drink colas because we're at a movie theater. We eat hors d'oeuvres because we're at a party. When we eat out of habit instead of hunger, it's almost a guarantee that we're eating calories in excess of our needs.

Depending on your body type, activity level and metabolism, you may need to eat only one large meal a day, or up to five smaller meals. Grazing—eating small portions of calorie-conscious foods every couple of hours—is a great way for some women to lose weight. It can maintain your blood sugar level, which will keep you from feeling "starved." Grazing may also help improve digestion for some individuals.

■ Eat Slowly

Along with making mealtime an activity unto itself, you can reduce the amount of food you consume by eating slowly. This will let the brain recognize the signals from the stomach so that you will feel full sooner on less food.

■ Drink Lots of Water

Water contains no calories, but it's absolutely essential to your well-being. Whatever diet you follow, supplement your meals with lots of water to aid digestion and help promote a feeling of fullness. Some people have a difficult time distinguishing between thirst and hunger, and you may find a glass of cool water satisfies that urge to indulge. Also, sodas and juices can contribute a substantial amount of calories to your diet. Replacing other liquids with calorie-free water is a simple way to cut back on total calories consumed.

Advanced Exercises

*W*hew! You've done it!

After completing week 16 of level three you should be feeling so good about the changes you've experienced that you're ready to do it all again! That's what the program is set up for: all you do is repeat the 16-week program, with additional resistance where you need it.

You're also going to need some new exercises to create additional challenges for the new strength you've developed. Some of these exercises have already been referenced in the last few weeks of the program for those of you go-getters who just can't wait.

You are now familiar with many exercises and with how your body changes and adapts to exercise. I can't speak for you about the additional changes you want to see in your body, but perhaps you want a little more muscular definition in your arms and

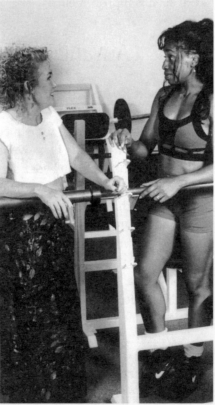

Tatiana was one of the first personal trainers certified in my Freestyle method. Today she is my top LBS trainer and also integral in the development of my new video series.

shoulders, or maybe a little more curve to your rear. This is where personal trainers become so valuable in helping people fine-tune their workouts and build the body of their dreams.

To help you, I've turned to one of my top personal trainers, Tatiana Byrne. "Tat" has been working with my programs for more than three years. She not only teaches the method, but because she is geographically close to me, we have also been working together to develop new exercises and programs. One of our most exciting projects is the *Lower Body Solution* video series.

Tatiana is a full-time personal trainer. While she never cared for bodybuilding, she has been an avid fan and competitor in fitness contests. The aspect she loves best is the performance, although she says the contests first inspired her to try my *Freestyle* methods.

"I was in the gym too much and getting more muscular than I wanted," she says.

To cut down the muscle she

began *Freestyle* in her own workouts, and then with her clients. It wasn't until one of her clients moved to the Napa Valley that she decided to venture to my small town. That's where we met in person, and I must say, I ran into one of my biggest fans.

Tatiana loves what she does with a passion and dedication that I rarely see. She is not only working with me on the video series, it was inspired by her high-energy body-sculpting classes. The professionalism and enthusiasm she brings to her work is why she is able to make a full-time living at personal training. She's good.

In this, our final chapter, Tatiana demonstrates some of the advanced moves that will help you continue to progress and prosper on the *Lower Body Solution* training program.

Use these exercises instead of some of the simpler versions in the level three routines. For example, replace the lunges and squats with the more difficult versions here. Add some of the other exercises, such as the biceps curl with a barbell for more arm definition, or the military press with a barbell for more shoulder emphasis.

Be creative. You've learned the sound principles of *Lower Body Solution* weight training for women. Now stick with the program and keep seeing improvements!

Advanced Exercise Index

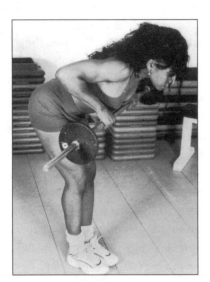

Bent-Over Row, Barbell
(middle back, shoulders)

Here's a great exercise to help correct rounded shoulders. When properly performed, the bent-over row will work the muscles of the middle back that help pull your shoulders back.

Grasp a barbell with an overhand grip (palms facing you), hands shoulder-width apart. Bend your knees and lean forward from the hips until your back is at a 45-degree angle to the floor. Keep your head in line with your spine or held slightly up, whichever is more comfortable, and arch your back. From this starting position, pull the bar to the middle of your chest, then slowly return to the start.

This should be a natural movement, using the muscles of the back and arms simultaneously.

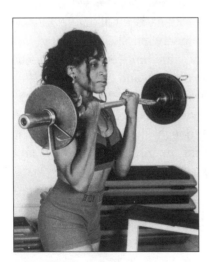

Biceps Curl, Barbell
(biceps)

Grasp a barbell with an underhand grip (palms facing away from your body). This hand position emphasizes the biceps, whereas performing the exercise with an overhand grip (palms facing the body) emphasizes the forearms. Stand with the barbell resting on your thighs.

Keeping your upper arms close to your sides and motionless during the exercise, slowly curl the weight as high as possible and then slowly lower to the start. Be careful not to hyperextend the elbows.

Throughout the exercise keep your head level, chest up, and chin retracted—there is a tendency to lean forward and poke your chin out as your muscles fatigue, so be aware of these posture tips. Also, do not try to use your legs or back to assist with the exercise.

Good Morning
(low back, hamstrings, buttocks)

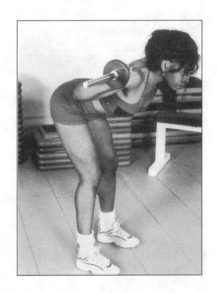

This exercise has been criticized because, if performed incorrectly or with too much weight, it can exacerbate lower-back injuries. However, when done correctly with light resistance, this is an excellent exercise for the hamstrings and glutes.

Stand with your feet shoulder-width apart and hold a lightweight bar across your shoulders. Flex your knees about 15 degrees and keep them unlocked throughout the exercise, as this will increase the involvement of your glutes and reduce the stress on your lower back. You should feel your bodyweight in the middle of your feet.

Keeping your head in line with your spine and your back slightly arched (neutral spine position), bend from the hips until you feel your bodyweight shift to the balls of your feet, which should occur at about 45 degrees. At this point your back should still be arched—if it is straight or rounded, you've gone too far. Return to the start to complete the exercise, but do not straighten so quickly that you hyperextend your back.

To increase the stability of your back while performing this exercise, hold your breath before you bend forward. Exhale only when you feel the weight shift off the balls of your feet as you rise.

If this exercise causes you back pain, substitute the back extension on a hyperextension bench. Back pain may also be a sign of a potentially chronic injury—check with a doctor to be safe.

Gorsha Lunge, Dumbbells
(thighs, buttocks, hamstrings)

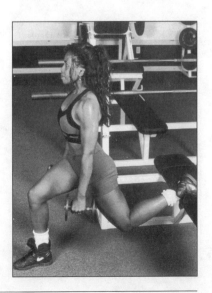

This exercise is similar to the stationary lunge, the difference being your rear leg is elevated to knee level. This distinction increases the stress on the working leg; thus, considerably less weight can be used on it when compared to other lunges.

Begin the exercise with your feet hip-width apart, torso erect and head level, holding two light dumbbells. Take a slow, controlled step forward with one leg, pointing it straight ahead or slightly out. Place the foot of the other leg on a chair behind you set at knee height. This is the start position for the exercise. Now lower your hips and allow your trailing knee to drop as far as comfortable. At its fullest stretch, your forward knee will be ahead of your ankle. Return to the start by flexing both legs simultaneously until they are straight.

Because there is less stability in this exercise compared to a stationary lunge, using a barbell is not recommended without spotters (preferably two, one on each side).

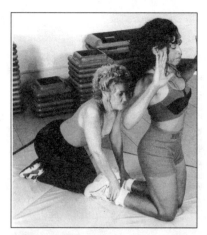

Harrop Hamstrings
(upper hamstrings, buttocks)

Here's one you won't see in most exercise books, but it is one of the most intense exercises for the glutes and hamstrings you can perform and should be a part of your *Lower Body Solution* training arsenal.

The hamstrings have two functions, to extend the hip and to flex the knee. This exercise works the hip extension function, which I like to refer to anatomically as the upper hamstrings. When describing exercises that flex the knee, we'll call those lower-hamstring exercises.

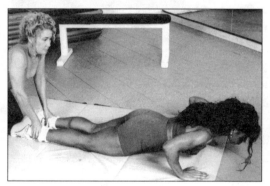

The Harrop Hamstrings requires someone to hold your feet, unless you can find a sturdy object to anchor your legs. You will also need a thick pad or towel, as it requires you to exercise from a kneeling position.

Kneel down and have your spotter anchor your lower legs by holding down your ankles—and he or she really needs to hold you down! Lift your hips up so your upper legs are in line with your torso. Now position your hands in front of you, arms slightly bent and elbows up, as if you were performing a push-up. This is the start position.

Keeping your legs and back aligned, slowly lower your body to the floor, allowing your arms to break your fall. As soon as you stop your momentum, vigorously push yourself back with your arms, contracting your glutes and hamstrings as you do so. Try not to bend at the waist during the exercise.

This is a tough exercise, so go easy on it for the first several workouts. Also, if you're especially weak in this area, you can modify the exercise by placing a sturdy bench in front of you to decrease the range of motion. As you progress, use a lower bench or step. Be patient; progress will come.

Jackknife Sit-Up
(upper abdominals)

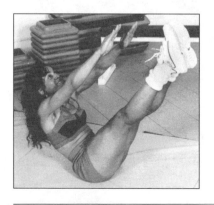

This exercise is commonly used by gymnasts. It combines a sit-up movement with an advanced leg lift so you can touch your toes while balancing on your glutes.

The jackknife is an advanced upper-abdominal exercise, and it should only be performed by those who have developed strong lower abdominal muscles. If this exercise bothers your back, it may be because you lack sufficient lower-abdominal (external obliques) strength to counter the pull of the hip flexor muscles. If this is the case, substitute easier upper-abdominal exercises such as the abdominal crunch.

Lower Body Solution Glute Blaster
(buttocks, hamstrings)

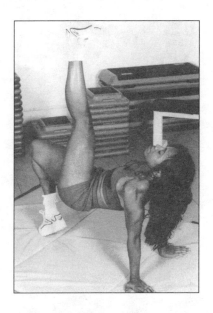

I consider this an advanced exercise because it so intensely targets your glutes and hamstrings.

Sit down with your legs in front of you, hands on the floor by your hips. Bend your right knee and place your foot flat on the floor. Keeping your left leg straight, raise it until it is perpendicular to the floor; as you do this, also lift your hips until they are at least parallel to the floor. Complete the movement by lifting your right heel off the floor and tilting your head back until you can see the ceiling. Now lower to the start. Perform all the reps for one side before switching legs.

Although most women will find just lifting their bodyweight sufficient resistance, you can increase the difficulty by using ankle weights.

Lunge/Curl Combination
(thighs, hamstrings, buttocks, biceps)

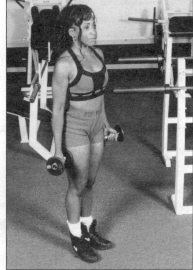

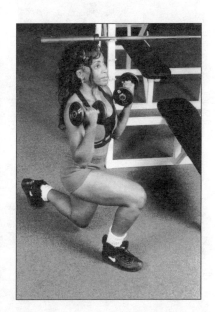

This is a great time-saver and calorie burner. Be certain that you are proficient in performing the forward lunge without a support for balance before you try it.

Hold a dumbbell in each hand. Begin with your feet nearly hip-width apart and your torso erect, and look straight ahead or slightly up. Take a big step forward and lower your hips, allowing your trailing knee to drop to a point just before it touches the floor. As you step forward, simultaneously curl the dumbbells to your upper arms. To return to the start, push off with your forward leg and then step back while lowering the dumbbells back to the start position. Repeat for the opposite leg. A single repetition for the lunge consists of one complete movement for each leg.

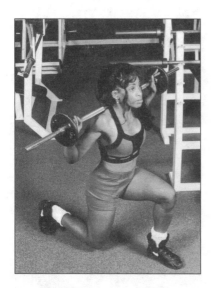

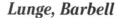

Lunge, Barbell

(thighs, hamstrings, buttocks)

To increase the difficulty of a lunge you can place a barbell behind your head, resting it on your shoulders, as shown. Never rest a barbell on your neck or cover the barbell with a thick towel, as this creates an unnatural stress on your neck.

Begin with your feet nearly hip-width apart and your torso erect. Look straight ahead or slightly up. Take a big step forward and lower your hips, allowing your trailing knee to drop to a point just before it touches the floor (never, ever, allow the knee to touch the floor). To return to the start, push off with your forward leg and then step back when the front knee is completely straight. Repeat for the opposite leg. A single repetition for the lunge consists of one complete movement for each leg.

Because your back is held vertical during this exercise, you should not feel any significant pressure on your lower back. If you do, you're probably leaning forward.

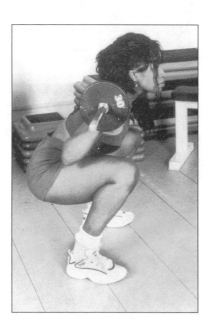

Squat, Barbell

(hips, thighs, buttocks)

The squat is an excellent exercise for the entire lower body and is very safe. Begin with a bar resting across your shoulders. Be sure you perform this in a safety cage or use a spotter. With your feet placed flat on the floor, shoulder-width apart, find a point high on the wall near the ceiling and focus your eyes on it. Rotate your elbows forward so they are perpendicular to the floor. This is your start position.

Keeping your head up and your torso as erect as possible (and only bending forward when absolutely necessary to drop further down), slowly bend your knees, allowing your knees to travel outward over your toes. Try to lower yourself so your thighs go well past parallel to the floor, but do not bottom out or bounce in the low position. Using your legs and resisting the temptation to lean forward excessively, push out of the bottom position to return to the start.

Squat Jump
(hips, thighs, glutes)

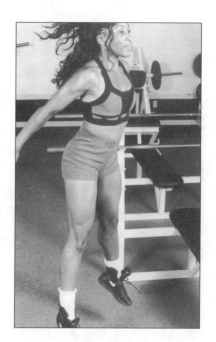

Jumping exercises provide a refreshing variety to your workouts. Jumping can be an intense training method, so you should probably avoid this exercise if you have a history of knee problems.

To perform them, it's important to have sturdy shoes, such as crosstrainers. Also, the surface you perform them on should be soft, such as an exercise mat or, if you exercise outdoors, grass or other groundcover.

This type of jump emphasizes the lower body in that the arms are primarily used for balance. Begin by lifting your arms in front of you and bending your knees. Now vigorously jump into the air and pull your arms down. As you land, flex your knees and lift your arms up again. Repeat for the required number of reps, performing the exercise in a fluid, rhythmical pattern.

Step-Up, Dumbbells
(thighs)

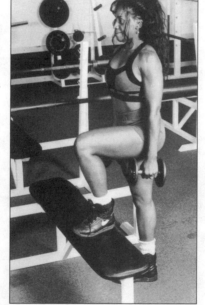

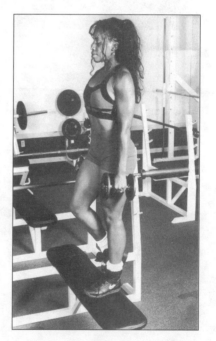

As you become stronger with the *Lower Body Solution*, you'll find that you will need to perform the step-up exercise with dumbbells.

Find a box (or several aerobic steps) high enough so that when you put one foot on it, your upper thigh is parallel to the floor. Hold two dumbbells at your sides with your palms facing each other. Position yourself facing the box so that the entire surface of your right foot is on the box and your left foot is on the floor, just a few inches away from the box. Point your right foot straight ahead or slightly out, whichever position you find the most stable. Pull your shoulders back and look straight ahead. This is the start position.

Perform the exercise by straightening your right leg, keeping your left foot just a few inches from the box. After straightening your right leg, slowly return to the start. Do not allow your back leg to cross behind your right as this will cause you to lose balance. Continue in this manner until you have completed all the reps for that side, then switch legs.

If you feel off-balance during this exercise, step onto the box at the top of each rep.

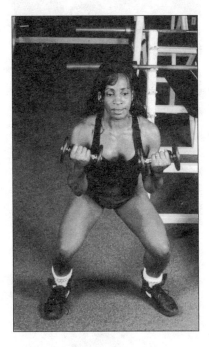
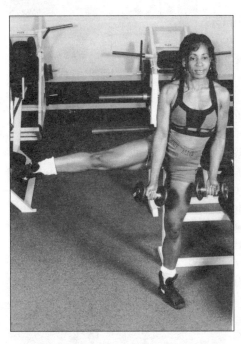

The "Tat" Squat
(thighs, hamstrings, buttocks, outer thighs)

This combines a dumbbell squat with a side leg raise, thereby increasing the work on the outer thigh and increasing the calorie-burning effects. This is one of Tatiana's favorite exercises and is named after her.

Begin with your feet nearly hip-width apart and torso erect. Look straight ahead or slightly up. Holding two dumbbells as shown, squat down as far as comfortable, keeping your back straight. Return to the top position. Now lift your right leg out to the side and lower slowly. Repeat the squat and kick out with the opposite leg. A single repetition is completed when you have completed a leg lift for each side.

This exercise takes a bit of practice to get comfortable with, so be patient. Also, as you progress, increase the difficulty by holding weights at your sides during the lunge and in front of your hips during the leg raise.

Exercise Index

A generation ago most of us were happy to own a color TV, an eight-track, and to watch *Happy Days*. Then came VCRs, cassette tapes and MTV. Now there's DVDs, CDs, and pay-per-view. Just as the entertainment industry has changed, the fitness industry has also evolved with sophisticated resistance training machines to help us get fit fast.

There is an ongoing debate in academic circles as to which is better, free weights or machines, but the fact is exercise machines do offer several advantages over free weights. For example, most contain selectorized weight stacks that enable you to change resistance in a few seconds by simply moving a pin. For those who are on a tight schedule, or are using a training protocol that requires minimal rest time between sets, this is a key benefit. Other machines, with their various pulley and lever-arm designs, can help you isolate particularly troublesome body parts. For example, the popular multi-hip machines enable you to isolate the inner and outer thighs. And with the advent of gravity-assisted chin-up and dip machines, all women can perform these effective exercises without having the strength of Xena, Warrior Princess. But probably the most impor-

tant benefits of exercise machines are that they provide variety to keep us motivated and are easy to use.

Whether you're using free weights or machines, to ensure maximum safety you must pay careful attention to technique. One problem with machines is that the design and performance varies with the manufacturer, so that 50 pounds on a Cybex leg curl may equal 70 pounds on a Nautilus. Whenever you're using a new machine, or if you have a question about how to perform a specific free-weight exercise, it's wise to ask an instructor for help. Although other gym members may be willing to offer advice, they may not know much more than you and could end up giving you poor advice.

To help you get the most out of your workouts, the following pages contain photos of each exercise used in the *Lower Body Solution*, along with detailed instructions. However, if you find that any exercise causes pain, don't do it! Simply substitute another exercise for the same bodypart. To help you with this I've listed the major muscles that each exercise works. But also consider that pain may indicate a hidden problem which may require medical attention, especially if other exercises for that same muscle group cause discomfort.

Demonstrating the exercises is elite U.S. figure skater and professional model, Veronica Chojnacki.

Abdominal Crunch

(upper abdominals)

This exercise isolates the upper abdominals far better than the conventional sit-up, which primarily works the hip flexor muscles that lift the legs.

Assume the start position with your hands cradling your jaw as shown, elbows tucked in against your chest. Besides helping to keep your head aligned with your spine, positioning the elbows down in this manner reduces the stress on your neck.

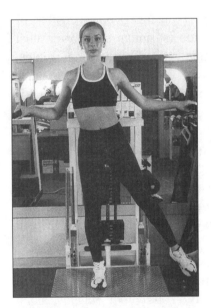

Perform the crunch by taking a breath, holding it, then curling your trunk to the point where the shoulder blades begin to lift off the floor. Exhale as you return to the start. Be certain to let your shoulders and head make full contact with the mat before performing another repetition; this technique enables you to work the muscles through a greater range of motion and further reduces the stress on your neck.

To make the exercise even more difficult, elevate your heels on a low step (about six inches), point your toes and press your heels against the surface of the step as you crunch. Pressing the heels down contracts the hamstrings, which in turn relaxes the hip flexors so your upper abs must work even harder.

Abduction, Multi-Hip Machine

(leg abductors)

Abduction is the act of moving your legs away from the midline of your body, so this type of machine is often called an abductor machine. This exercise can be performed on either a standing multi-hip machine or a seated abductor machine. Whichever you choose, follow the instructions on the machine as these vary with the manufacturer.

With the multi-hip machine, you will perform abduction with the pad on the outside of the thigh. Align your hips with the center of the pulley and point your foot straight ahead. Begin the exercise by lifting your free leg out to the side as far as comfortable, being careful not to arch your back or rotate your hips. Slowly return to the start. Complete all the repetitions for that leg before switching to the other leg.

When you use the seated version, your back and hips should always remain in contact with the backrest; use a seatbelt if one is provided. Without lifting your hips or leaning forward, spread your legs apart slowly—do not jerk the weight (which is easy to do on this exercise because many machines have some slack in the cable) as this could strain your lower back. When your legs are opened as far as comfort allows, slowly return to the start.

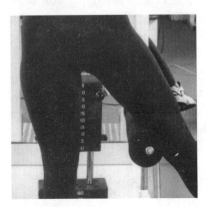

If an abductor machine is not available, you can perform this exercise with a low-pulley unit. This entails attaching the cable to one ankle, standing so your non-working leg is closest to the weight stack, and then lifting your free leg away from the weight stack.

Adduction, Multi-Hip Machine

(leg adductors)

Adduction is the act of pulling your legs toward the midline of your body, so this type of machine is often called an adductor machine. This exercise can be performed on either a standing multi-hip machine or a seated adductor machine. Whichever you choose, follow the instructions on the machine as these vary with the manufacturer.

If using a multi-hip machine, stand so your hips are aligned with the center of the pulley. Adjust the pad so it rests on the middle portion of one of your inner thighs,

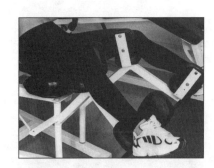

not on your knee. Point your foot straight ahead, not out. Without rotating your hips or leaning forward, allow the lever arm to swing as high as comfortable. Without jerking the weight, slowly pull your leg toward your body until it is perpendicular to the ground (or slightly crossing the other leg if the design of the machine permits). Perform all the reps for that leg before switching to the other leg.

If using the seated version, your back and hips should always remain in contact with the backrest; use a seatbelt if one is provided. Without lifting your hips or leaning forward, close your legs together slowly—do not jerk the weight (which is easy to do on this exercise because many machines have some slack in the cable) as this could strain your lower back. When your legs are pulled together as close as possible, slowly return to the start.

If an adductor machine is not available, you can perform this exercise with a low-pulley unit. This entails attaching the cable to your ankle, standing so your working leg is closest to the weight stack (you'll have to stand several feet away from the machine so that the working leg is pulled away from the body and experiences resistance), and then lifting your free leg away from the weight stack.

Back Extension

(lower back)

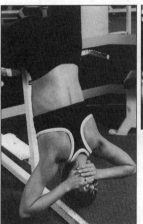

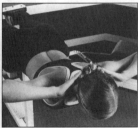

Lie facedown on a hyperextension bench and lock your ankles in place (or hook them under the roller pad if a footrest is not available). Adjust your hips on the pad so that when you bend forward your back is perpendicular to the floor but not rounded—this is the start position. Put your hands on the sides of your head and, keeping your head in alignment with your spine (which entails retracting your chin and not looking up), lift your torso until your back is parallel to the floor. Slowly return to the start. Lifting your torso higher than parallel is unnecessary and may place harmful stress on the back.

To increase the resistance, you can place a medicine ball or weight plate behind your upper back, just below the base of your neck. Do not place weights on your head or neck, as this could result in injury. Another way to increase resistance is to hold a weight plate or medicine ball on your chest, crossing your arms to secure it.

Bench Press, Barbell

(pectorals, anterior deltoids, triceps)

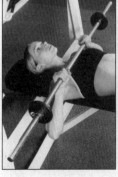

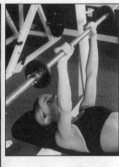

The bench press is unquestionably the most popular upper-body weight training exercise because it involves all the upper-body pushing muscles. However, it should not be performed with heavy weights, or too frequently, as it could develop pectoral muscles that appear square, like a man's.

Lie faceup on a bench press unit, straddling the bench and spreading your legs shoulder-width apart, feet flat on the floor. If your feet don't touch the floor, place weight plates under your heels—this will prevent you from arching your back. Grasp the barbell with a shoulder-width grip and have a spotter help you position the weight at arms' length directly above your eyes. Take a deep breath, hold it, and slowly lower the weight to your mid- or lower chest, whichever is more comfortable. As you lower the weight, your elbows should point slightly down, not directly out to your sides. Without bouncing the barbell off your chest, press the weight back to the start, exhaling when your arms are nearly straight. When you've completed all your repetitions for a set, have your spotter help guide the barbell back to the supports.

I can't emphasize enough the importance of using a spotter when performing this exercise. The assistance of a spotter minimizes the stress that occurs to the smaller muscles of the shoulder when you remove or replace the barbell on the supports, and his or her presence is also essential for safety. Should you overestimate your strength and find yourself unable to remove the barbell from your chest, the spotter can remove it—otherwise, you would have to throw the weight to one side or roll it down your body; techniques that have been known to cause serious injury.

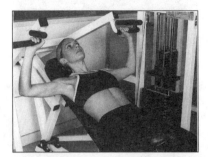

Bench Press, Incline Machine

(pectorals, anterior deltoids, triceps)

This machine lets you perform a bench press from a seated position so that instead of pushing the weight vertically, you push it horizontally. This design enables you to safely perform the exercise without a spotter.

Sit on the bench and place your feet flat on the floor. Grasp the handles with a shoulder-width grip. Take a deep breath, hold it, and press the weight to arms' length, keeping your elbows pointed slightly down, not directly out to your sides. Exhale as your arms lock out.

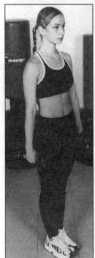

Biceps Curl, Dumbbells

(biceps)

Grasp two dumbbells and stand with your arms at your sides, palms facing forward. Keeping your upper arms close to your sides and motionless during the exercise, slowly curl the dumbbells as high as possible and then slowly lower to the start. Be careful not to hyperextend the elbows.

Throughout the exercise keep your head level, chest up, and chin retracted—there is a tendency to lean forward and poke your chin out as your muscles fatigue, so be aware of these posture tips. Also, do not try to use your legs or back to assist with the exercise. This exercise can also be performed on an incline bench with two dumbbells.

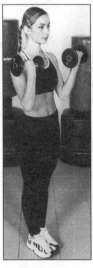
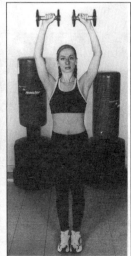

Biceps Curl with Shoulder Press

(biceps, shoulders)

This is a combination of two exercises, a biceps curl followed by a shoulder press. It is a very economical exercise from a time standpoint because it enables you to perform two exercises at once.

Grasp two dumbbells and stand with your arms at your sides, palms facing forward. Keeping your upper arms close to your sides, and motionless during the exercise, slowly curl the dumbbells as high as possible, then twist your hands away from your body and press the weights overhead and together. Slowly lower the weights to your shoulders and then back to your sides. This entire sequence equals one repetition.

Lower Body Solution

Cable Crunch
(upper abdominals)

This exercise requires access to a high-pulley apparatus and a rope attachment. This is a variation of the crunch that enables you to incrementally increase the resistance.

Hook the rope attachment to the high pulley. Grasp the rope handles and turn your back to the machine. Get on your knees, but lift your hips so they do not touch your hamstrings. From this start position, hold your breath and crunch forward without moving your legs. Exhale as you slowly return to the start.

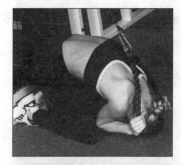

Calf Raise, Seated
(lower calf)

This exercise adds shape to the lower portion of the calf muscle called the soleus. Training the soleus improves ankle stability, an important factor in *Lower Body Solution* training because of its emphasis on lunge exercises.

Sit on a seated calf bench with your toes facing forward. Adjust the weight or padded bar just behind your knees; placing the weight on the knees could injure your kneecaps. To ensure a complete range of motion of the soleus, you must position your foot so you can drop your heels below the balls of your feet. Begin the exercise by lowering your heels below your toes as far as comfortable, then raise them as high as possible. Pause at this peak contraction position before slowly lowering to the start.

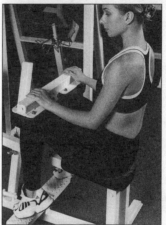

You might feel a slight burning sensation while performing this exercise, which is perfectly normal. Also, because this exercise has the potential to make your calves especially sore, for your first several workouts you should use light weights.

Calf Raise, Standing
(calves)

Position yourself on a standing calf machine by placing your feet so your heels can extend below the toes; this will enable you to get a full stretch on the muscles. With your legs straight, lower your heels as far as comfortable and then raise your heels as high as possible to achieve maximum contraction. Pause momentarily in this position before slowly lowering to the stretched position. Foot position can be varied to change the emphasis.

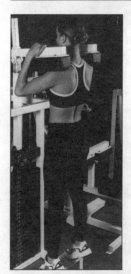

You might feel a slight burning sensation while performing this exercise, which is perfectly normal. Also, because this exercise has the potential to make your calves especially sore, for your first several workouts you should use light weights.

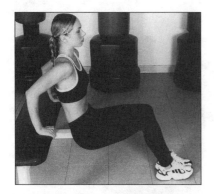

Chair Dip

(triceps, pectorals, anterior deltoids)

Place two sturdy benches about three feet apart. Position yourself so your back is to one bench with your hands grasping the edge of the bench. Your arms should be straight and your elbows pointed back. Rest your heels on the floor. Begin the exercise by bending your arms as far as comfortable and then straightening them to return to the start. To increase the difficulty, rest your heels on a higher bench or have a spotter place weight plates across your hips.

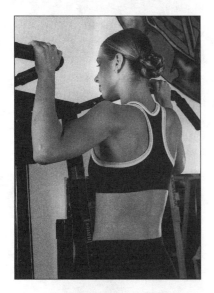

Chin-Up Machine

(upper back)

This exercise works the muscles of the upper back called the latissimus dorsi, or lats. With the chin-up, your palms face you; with a pull-up, your palms face away from you. The chin-up is usually easier to perform as the biceps have better leverage to pull from.

Because many women have difficulty performing chin-ups and pull-ups, I recommend performing this exercise on a Gravitron or similar machine. These machines allow you to offset your bodyweight. For example, a 140-pound woman can reduce the weight she lifts by a percentage, say 50 percent, and perform the exercise with only 70 pounds instead of 140 pounds. Since each machine is different, you should follow the directions provided on the unit you are using.

Begin the chin-up by grasping the chinning bar and placing your legs on the support platform. Simultaneously flex your arms and pull your shoulders down until your chin is level with the bar (or slightly lower if you find the former range of motion uncomfortable). Now slowly lower yourself to the start, being careful not to hyperextend your arms at the finish. When you've completed the exercise, step off the platform, using your arms for support, then let go of the bar.

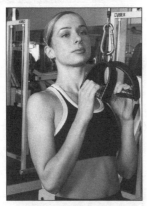

Close-Grip Pulldown, Parallel Grip

(upper back, biceps)

This variation of the pulldown is performed with your hands facing each other, spaced about eight inches apart. It requires the use of a V-handle attachment, which is available in most health clubs.

Sit on a lat pulldown machine so your torso is positioned slightly behind the cable. Begin by pulling the bar to the upper portion of your chest, leaning slightly back as you do so. Pause in this fully contracted position and then slowly return to the start. This should be a natural movement, using the muscles of the back and arms simultaneously.

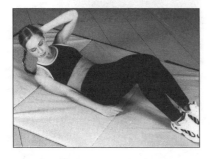

Cross Crunch

(obliques, upper abdominals)

This abdominal exercise is a variation of the crunch that works not only the upper abdominals but also the obliques.

Place your right hand on the side of your head, just behind the ear, and cross your left leg over your right. Hold your breath, curl forward and twist your head, neck and shoulders as a unit to bring your right elbow to your left knee. Slowly return to the start position. After you've completed all the reps for that side, reverse the movement for the abdominal muscles on the other side of the trunk.

The exercise is considered complete when you fully contract the obliques, which may not require touching an elbow to knee. To more effectively isolate the upper abdominals, drape your lower legs over the top of a bench so your upper legs are perpendicular to the floor.

During this exercise do not tuck your chin against your chest; instead, leave a few inches of space between your jaw and collarbone. When you return to the start, let your shoulders and head make full contact with the mat before performing another repetition. This ensures that the muscles are worked through a full range of motion and minimizes the stress on the neck and upper back.

Crunch Machine
(upper abdominals)

This exercise can be performed on a variety of apparatus, and is reserved for intermediate and advanced trainees.

Regardless of the machine you use, perform the crunch by holding your breath, curling your shoulders and "crunching" on the abdominal muscles. When you return to the start, let your shoulders and head come back to the neutral position before performing another repetition.

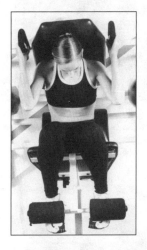

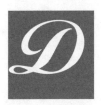

Deadlift, Dumbbell
(legs, lower back)

Although this exercise is often considered primarily a back exercise, it is also an effective lower-body exercise because the legs work through a wide range of motion.

Position yourself for this exercise by straddling a dumbbell. Spread your feet shoulder-width apart and point your feet slightly out, in line with your knees. Stand the dumbbell on one end and grasp the plates on the other side with both hands. Arch your back and look straight ahead or slightly up; this is the start position.

Perform the exercise by straightening your legs and then your back until you reach a fully upright position. Keeping your head in the same position and your back arched, slowly reverse the movement until the weight touches the floor. Throughout this exercise keep the dumbbell close to the body, as this will minimize the stress on your lower back.

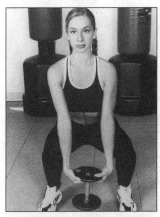

Dip, Machine
(triceps, shoulders, chest)

This is an excellent compound movement for the upper-body pushing muscles: triceps, shoulders and chest.

Because many women have difficulty performing dips, I recommend performing this exercise on a Gravitron or similar machine. These machines allow you to offset your bodyweight. For example, a 140-pound woman can reduce the weight she lifts by a percentage, say 50 percent, and perform the exercise with only 70 pounds instead of 140 pounds. Since each machine is different, you should follow the directions provided on the unit you are using.

Begin the dip by grasping the dip handles and placing your legs on the support platform. Your wrists should be straight, in line with your forearms. Simultaneously bend your arms and, while slightly leaning forward, lower yourself as for as comfortable, then lengthen your arms to return to the start. Do not hyperextend your arms at the finish. When you've completed the exercise, step off the platform, using your arms for support, then let go of the handles.

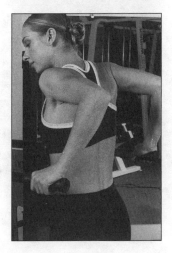

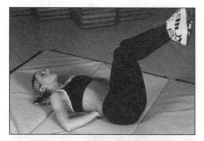

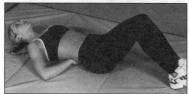

Double Leg Lowering
(lower abs)

After you master the pelvic tilt, this is a good exercise to use to further strengthen the lower abdominals. It requires no special equipment other than a soft surface such as an exercise mat.

Lie faceup and place your hands underneath your lower back. Pull your knees to your chest, tucking your ankles against your buttocks. From this starting position, slowly lower your legs to the floor without straightening your legs or arching your back. To ensure that your back is not arching, press your lower back against your arms.

As you master this exercise, increase the difficulty by straightening your legs.

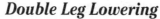

Hip Extension, Multi-Hip Machine
(upper hamstrings)

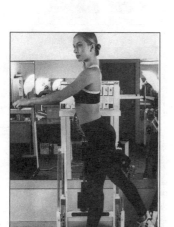

Here's another exercise that works the hip extension function of the hamstrings:

Stand facing sideways to the machine so your hips are aligned with the center of the pulley. Adjust the pad so it rests on the middle portion of one of your hamstrings, not on your knee. Point your foot straight ahead, not out. Without rotating your hips or leaning forward, allow the lever arm to swing as high as comfortable, then slowly push the weight down and back as far as possible in the other direction. Do not jerk the weight, as this could strain your back and hamstrings. Repeat with the other leg.

If this machine is not available, you can perform a similar exercise with a low-pulley machine. Attach a cable ankle strap to your leg and hook it to the cable. Stand facing the machine, and step back about two feet so you can move the working leg forward with resistance. With the working leg outstretched, lift it backward in an arch as high as comfortable without leaning forward or turning your hips. Return to the start and repeat.

Horse Stance
(lower back, upper back)

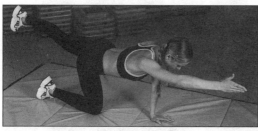

This is a great exercise to improve your posture. It strengthens the spinae erectors, the two cable-like muscles that run down the middle of your back, and many of the small postural muscles of the upper back and neck.

Get down on all fours (knees and palms) so your upper thighs and your arms are perpendicular to the floor. Your hands should be directly under your shoulders and your elbows pointed back. Bend your arms so your upper back is parallel to the floor. Your head should be aligned with your spine—do not look up! This is the start position.

Begin the exercise by lifting and extending your right arm in front of you until it is parallel to the floor. Turn your hand so your thumb is pointing up. Now extend and lift your left leg until it is also parallel to the floor. Hold this position for the required number of seconds, then perform the same movement with the left arm and the right leg. Continue alternating sides in this manner for the prescribed number of repetitions.

Because this exercise involves many smaller postural muscles, and because postural muscles must contract for extended periods, the workouts prescribed have you holding each position for extended periods (often up to 30 seconds). You'll find that when you first perform this exercise, trying to hold the positions for more than just a few seconds is quite a struggle. Also, you'll notice that one side of your body is usually much more stable than the other—this is perfectly normal and is often simply a result of daily lifestyle postures that create muscle imbalances.

Lateral Raise
(shoulders)

Hold two light dumbbells at your sides, palms facing each other. Keep your elbows slightly bent, knees unlocked, and look straight ahead. Using just the strength of your shoulders, slowly pull the weights upward until they are perpendicular to the floor, no higher, and then return to the start.

Avoid the tendency to arch your back and look up while performing this exercise. Besides placing harmful stress on your spine, this faulty stance will not adequately emphasize the muscles you want to work during this exercise. If you have trouble maintaining correct posture, or cannot lift the weights high enough, you're probably using weights that are simply too heavy.

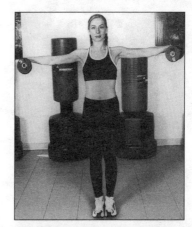

Leg Curl, Prone and Seated
(hamstrings)

There are several types of leg curl machines available, but the two most common are those that allow you to perform the exercise prone (facedown) and those that allow you to perform the exercise seated. The advantage of the seated machines is they remove any potential strain on your lower back; with the prone leg curl machines, there is a tendency to arch your back. The basic techniques for using these machines, however, are the same.

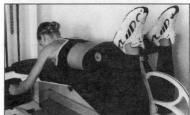

Regardless of the type of machine you have access to, you want to position yourself so your ankles rest behind the pads. On the prone leg curl machines your knees should extend at least an inch beyond the bench (to avoid compressing your kneecaps), and on both machines you want to have your knees in line with the pulley (cam). Also, always keep your toes pointed so your calves don't cramp and to increase the emphasis on the hamstrings.

Begin the exercise by slowly pulling your ankles toward your buttocks; ideally, you want the pad to touch your buttocks. Hold the peak contraction briefly before returning to the start position. Avoid the tendency to swing the weight; if you can't achieve a full range of motion without swinging, the weight you're using is probably too heavy.

It's important to achieve a full range of motion on this exercise. If you cannot do so, your hip flexors may be tight, the weight you are using may be too heavy, or the machine you are using may be poorly designed.

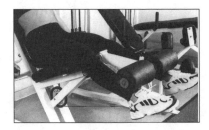

Leg Extension

(thighs)

This is an exercise that isolates the quadriceps. Because this movement places a high level of stress on the knees, it should only be used infrequently in your workouts. Exercises that are more "knee-friendly" include squats and step-ups.

Sit in a leg extension machine and grasp the handles to steady your torso. You should be positioned so the pads are directly behind your ankles; placing them over the top of your foot puts excessive pressure on your shins and knees. Raise the padded bar until your knees are straight (but not hyperextended), then slowly lower the weight to the start position.

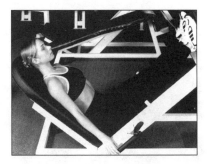

Leg Press Calf Raise

(calves)

Despite their relatively small size, the calves are capable of moving large weights in many exercises. The leg press machine significantly reduces the stress on your lower back when performing calf exercises, especially when compared to standing calf raises.

Position yourself on the machine by placing your feet so your heels can extend beyond the toes; this will enable you to get a full stretch on the muscles. Your back and head should be in contact with the backrest. With your legs straight, move your feet down the footrest so your heels extend over the edge. Begin the exercise by lowering your heels as far as comfortable and then raise up on the balls of your feet as high as possible. Repeat for the prescribed number of repetitions.

Because this exercise has the potential to make your calves especially sore, for your first several workouts you will want to use light weights. You might also experience a slight burning sensation in the calves when performing this exercise; this is perfectly normal and can be expected, especially when performing high reps.

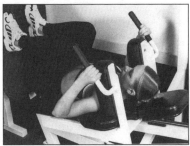

Leg Press, Horizontal

(quads, buttocks, hamstrings)

The leg press is a particularly effective leg exercise because it works all the major lower-body muscles through an extensive range of motion. In contrast to the leg extension exercise that isolates the quadriceps, the leg press also works the hamstrings and glutes.

Position yourself in the machine so your feet are flat on the footrest and your back and neck make full contact with the backrest. You should be sitting so your hips are not lifted off the backrest. Place your hands on the handles provided. From this start position, straighten your legs until they are straight but not hyperextended. Slowly return to the start.

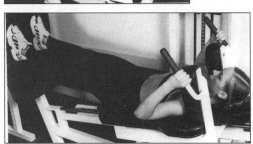

As you perform the exercise, be careful to avoid excessively arching or rounding the lower back. If you cannot avoid doing so, then the weight you are using is probably too heavy. The best leg press machines have a built-in lumbar support that minimizes the stress on the lower back. According to exercise scientist Dr. Mel Siff, if you are using a leg press machine that doesn't have a backrest that matches the natural curvature of your spine (a lumbar support), you can protect yourself by placing a small rolled-up towel under your lower back. The towel should be approximately the width and thickness of your fist, thereby helping to ensure the proper spinal posture when exerting maximum force with your legs.

Leg Press, Inclined
(quads, buttocks, hamstrings)

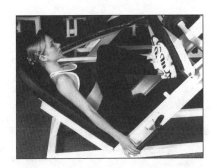

This is similar to the horizontal leg press, except you begin with your knees straight and you press the weights at an angle. Beginning with the legs straight tends to decrease the tendency to arch your back.

Position yourself in the machine so your feet are flat on the footrest and your back and neck make full contact with the backrest. Place your hands on the handles provided, then release the footrest supports. From this start position, straighten your legs until they are straight but not hyperextended. Slowly return to the start. When you've completed the set, lock in the safety support.

As you perform the exercise, be careful to avoid excessively arching or rounding the lower back. If you cannot avoid doing so, then the weight you are using is probably too heavy. As with the horizontal leg press, if the machine you are using doesn't have a lumbar support, place a small rolled-up towel under your lower back. The rolled-up towel should be approximately the width and thickness of your fist.

Lower Body Solution Lunges

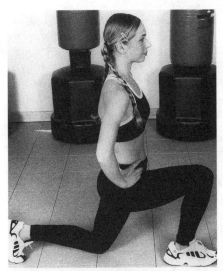

Lunge, Front
(thighs, hamstrings, buttocks)

Also known as the forward lunge, this exercise is performed with or without additional weight; you can hold dumbbells in each hand or place a barbell behind your head, resting it on your shoulders. Never rest a barbell on your neck or cover the barbell with a thick towel, as this creates an unnatural stress on the neck.

Begin with your feet nearly hip-width apart and your torso erect, and look straight ahead or slightly up. Take a big step forward and lower your hips, allowing your trailing knee to drop to a point just before it touches the floor (never, ever, allow the knee to touch the floor). To return to the start, push off with your forward leg and then step back when the front knee is completely straight. Repeat for the opposite leg. A single repetition for the lunge consists of one complete movement for each leg.

Because your back is held vertical during this exercise, you should not feel any significant pressure on your lower back. If you do, you're probably leaning forward during the exercise or have weak back muscles, which should tone up significantly after a few weeks on the *Lower Body Solution*.

Other variations of the lunge include:

Lunge, Bench on Smith Machine
(quadriceps, hamstrings, buttocks)

This variation of the lunge is performed on a Smith machine and requires a step or platform about four to six inches high. A step will enable you to achieve a greater range of motion during this exercise, thus increasing the calorie-burning effects.

Place the step about a foot in front of the machine and position yourself on the machine with the bar on the back of your shoulders. Keeping your torso erect and your head level, place one foot on the platform and step back about two to three feet (depending upon flexibility) with the other. This is your start position.

Begin the exercise by lowering your hips so your forward thigh drops below parallel with the floor. At the fullest stretch, your forward knee will be positioned slightly ahead of your ankle, with your foot pointing straight ahead or slightly out (whichever position you find the most stable). Complete the movement by straightening both legs. Continue lunging in this manner until you have completed all the reps for that leg. When finished, bring your legs together, step forward with the other leg, and perform an equal number of repetitions for that leg.

Make certain the bench or step you use is stable—it must not slide during the exercise. Also, some gyms have angled boxes that you can use to perform this exercise and that will reduce the stress on the ankles and knees. Experiment to determine what is best for you.

Lunge, Gorsha
(thighs, hamstrings, buttocks)

This exercise is similar to the stationary lunge, the difference is your rear leg is elevated to knee level. This distinction increases the stress on the working leg; thus, considerably less weight can be used on it when compared to other lunges. I first heard about the exercise from Gorsha Sur, a former U.S. National Champion in ice dancing.

Begin the exercise with your feet hip-width apart, torso erect and head level. Take a slow, controlled step forward with one leg, pointing it straight ahead or slightly out. Place the foot of the other leg on a chair behind you set at knee height. This is the start position for the exercise. Now lower your hips and allow your trailing knee to drop as far as comfortable. At its fullest stretch, your forward knee will be ahead of your ankle. Return to the start by flexing both legs simultaneously until they are straight.

Resistance is usually increased by holding weights, as it is difficult to place a barbell on your back and get into position to perform it. Also, because there is less stability in this exercise compared to a stationary lunge, using a barbell is not recommended without spotters (preferably two, one on each side).

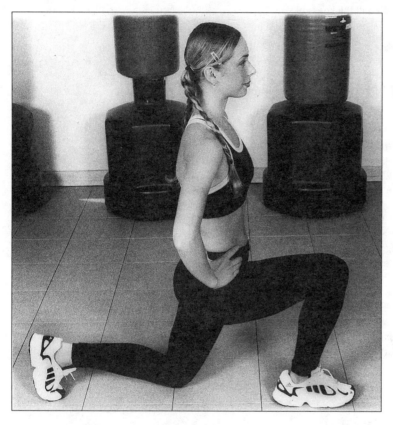

Lunge, Reverse
(thighs, hamstrings, buttocks)

This is one of the most neglected of the lunge series; but it is one of the most valuable, as it places minimal stress on the knees. Begin with your feet nearly shoulder-width apart, torso erect. Your front foot should be pointing straight ahead or slightly out, whichever position provides the most balance.

Begin by taking a slow, controlled step backward with one leg, lowering your hips so your forward thigh becomes parallel to the floor. Your knee should be positioned directly over your ankle and foot and your trailing knee extended to stretch your hip flexor muscles. The exertion phase of the exercise occurs when you push off your rear foot to return to the start position. Repeat for the opposite leg.

Lunge, Reverse, from Bench
(thighs, hamstrings, buttocks)

This is an excellent variation of the reverse lunge because it enables you to begin performing the movement through a greater range of motion. However, to perform it you need a stable low bench or step about four to six inches high. If you do not have such a platform, simply perform it without the step.

Stand on the platform with your feet nearly shoulder-width apart. You want your heels near the edge but still with both feet in full contact with the platform. Your front foot should be pointing straight ahead or slightly out, whichever position provides the most balance.

Begin by taking a slow, controlled step backward with one leg, lowering your hips so your forward thigh becomes parallel to the floor. Your knee should be positioned directly over your ankle and foot and your trailing knee extended to stretch your hip flexor muscles. The exertion phase of the exercise occurs when you push off your rear foot to return to the start position. Complete all the reps for that set before switching legs.

Lunge, Reverse, with Cable

(thighs, buttocks, extra emphasis on hamstrings)

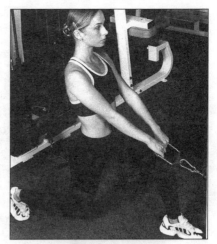

This is one of the most neglected of the lunge series; but because of its additional emphasis on the hamstrings, it is one of the most important. It requires a low pulley, such as the one found on a cable crossover machine.

While facing the weight stack, grasp the low-pulley handle with two hands and step back about two feet. Your arms should be straight. Spread your feet nearly shoulder-width apart, torso erect. Take a slow, controlled step backward with one leg, lowering your hips so your forward thigh becomes parallel to the floor. Your knee should be positioned directly over your ankle and foot. Your front foot should be pointing straight ahead and your trailing knee extended to stretch your hip flexor muscles. The exertion phase of the exercise occurs when you push off your rear foot and step back to return to the start position in one fluid motion. Repeat for the opposite leg.

Lunge, Side

(thighs, hamstrings, buttocks)

This lunge is performed by stepping out to the side. Make certain that the toe of your forward leg is pointed slightly outward. Allow the knee of your forward leg to extend directly over your forward foot, but not beyond your toes. Push yourself upright to the starting position. Repeat for the opposite leg. A single repetition for the lunge consists of one complete movement for each leg.

Lunge, Stationary

(thighs, hamstrings, buttocks)

This lunge is also very safe on the knees. It is sometimes referred to as a Split Squat. Take a large step forward. In this position, lower yourself until your trailing knee comes near the floor, then using your leg strength push yourself upright, but do not bring your legs together. Continue performing your repetitions in this manner until you have completed the set. Reverse forward legs, and perform the same repetitions for the opposite side.

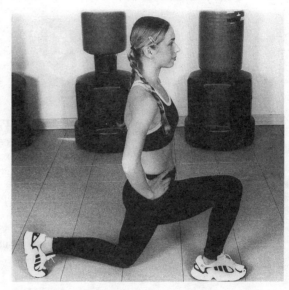

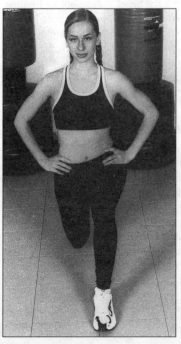

Lunge Walk

(thighs, hamstrings, buttocks)

Lunge walks should be done to fatigue without additional resistance. You'll need a large space, such as the perimeter of a gym or aerobics room.

Place your hands on your hips, and keep them there throughout the exercise. Using long, controlled steps, lunge forward, bending your front leg so the rear knee almost touches the floor. Recover by straightening your forward leg and bringing your rear leg up to meet your front leg. Repeat with the other leg, and continue alternating your legs in this walking motion. As you walk keep your torso erect and your head level.

When you first perform the exercise, walk near a wall so you can catch yourself if you lose your balance. As you progress, you can hold dumbbells at your sides to increase the difficulty.

Military Press, Dumbbells
(shoulders, triceps)

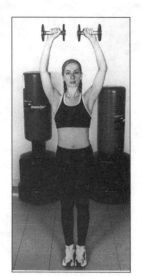

The military press is a gym standard because it provides excellent toning and strengthening effects to the shoulders and triceps.

Grasp a dumbbell in each hand and lift them to your shoulders, palms facing away from your body. Hold your breath and then press the dumbbells overhead to arms' length; the weights should travel in an arch, coming together at the top. Lower to complete the movement.

Do not at any point in the movement lean backward; this is a technique problem that can hurt the lower back. It is usually caused by using weights that are too heavy.

One-Arm Row, Dumbbell
(middle back, biceps)

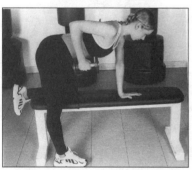

This is a great exercise for strengthening the back. Grasp a dumbbell with your right hand. Bend your left knee and rest it over a flat bench, your right foot on the floor, and your left arm on the bench. Bend forward from the waist so your back is parallel to the floor. Perform the exercise by pulling the dumbbell to the middle portion of your chest in one smooth motion, then slowly lowering to the start. Perform all the reps for that side before repeating for the other side.

If you have trouble holding on to the dumbbells during the exercise, use weightlifting gloves or straps to reinforce your grip.

One-Arm Row, Seated, with Cable
(middle back, biceps, obliques)

Although this is primarily an exercise for the middle back, the twisting that occurs during this exercise also affects the obliques and, to a small extent, even the lower back. It has been popularized by corrective exercise therapist Paul Chek in his seminars.

Sit in front of a low-pulley machine that has a swivel-mounted pulley. If this is not available, most cable crossover machines have this design. This is important, because with a fixed pulley the cable can easily slip over the groove of the pulley. Grasp a pulley handle with your left hand, palm down. Point your other hand straight ahead, parallel to the floor. This is the start position.

Begin by pulling the handle to the middle portion of your chest in one smooth motion, rotating your hand so your thumb is pointed up at the finish. As you do so, extend your other hand straight ahead so your body twists slightly. Slowly return the weight to the start, untwisting your hand as you do so. Perform all the reps for that set before repeating for the other side.

If you have trouble holding on to the cable during the exercise, use weightlifting gloves or straps to reinforce your grip.

Pec Dec
(chest)

The advantage of the pec dec is that it allows you to work the pectoral and shoulder muscles through an extensive range of motion.

Sit in the machine and align your shoulders with the center of the pulleys. Grasp the handles and rest your lower arms on the pads. Without jerking the weight, squeeze the handles together and then slowly allow them to return to the start.

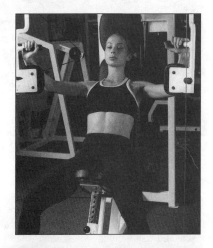

Pelvic Tilt
(lower abs)

Here's an isolation exercise for the lower abdominals that also helps stretch the lower back muscles.

Lie on your back, bend your knees, and place your arms behind your head. From this starting position, press your lower back into the floor, pulling in with the muscles of your lower abdomen so your hips roll under and upward. As you perform the movement, breathe in and out easily, keeping your neck and shoulders relaxed.

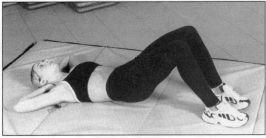

Once you've mastered this precise movement, work on performing the exercise with less bend in your knees. With practice, eventually you should be able to perform it with your knees almost straight. Repeat.

Petersen Step-Up
(quadriceps)

The Petersen step-up isolates the quadriceps muscle called the vastus medialis, a teardrop-shaped muscle on the inner thigh. Because this muscle is involved in knee stability, exercises such as the Petersen step-up are often used for knee rehabilitation. In fact, if you experience pain while performing lunges, often all it takes to resolve the problem is a few weeks performing the Petersen step-up.

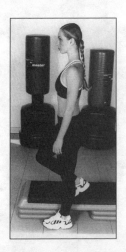

Straddle a low step, placing your left foot on the step and the right foot on the floor. Move your front leg back so the toes are just behind the heel of the foot on the floor. Now lift your right heel off the floor. This is the start position.

Perform the exercise by simultaneously straightening your right leg while pressing the heel to the floor, rocking back slightly as you do so. Slowly return to the start.

As you progress, you can raise the height of the bench and hold dumbbells while performing the exercise.

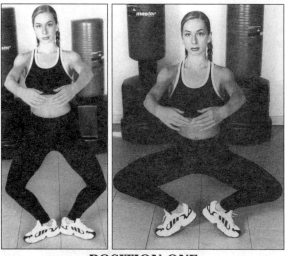

POSITION ONE

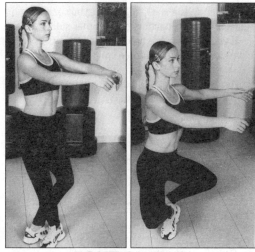

POSITION TWO

Plié

(thighs, hamstrings, buttocks)

This classic movement was developed in the 17th century for ballerinas. Pliés are excellent stretches and as performed in conjunction with the *Lower Body Solution* are great thigh toners as well. These exercises also contribute to balance and flexibility. If you are not familiar with the moves, begin with only a limited range of motion. Check the prescribed tempos—you will be lowering and rising much slower than when you perform the other exercises in this routine. Strive to keep your heels close to the floor; however, to enjoy maximum benefit from the stretch and toning action, you will need to raise your heels slightly to achieve a greater range of motion. To get into each of the positions you need to rotate the legs outward at the hip joint. This "turnout" will give you more flexibility in the hips. The arm motions are not necessary to the exercise, but assist your balance. There are actually five positions for the plié; we have modified four for this routine.

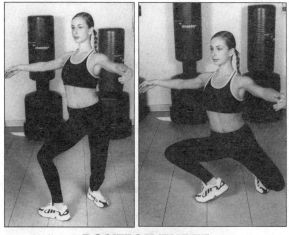

POSITION THREE

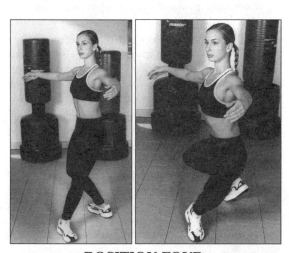

POSITION FOUR

Position One

Stand with your toes pointed out to the sides (as far as comfortable) and your heels about 18 inches apart. Bring your arms in front of you, forming a circle. Using your thigh muscles, slowly lower into a plié, making sure your knees extend over your toes. As you lower, bring your arms out to the sides. Rise from the plié bringing your arms back into a circle and bringing your legs together. (For variation, this can also be performed with your heels together.)

Position Two

An easier version of this can be done by placing the heel of your right foot against the middle of your left foot. Our model demonstrates a more advanced version whereby the right foot is placed parallel to the left foot, toe-to-heel and heel-to-toe. Using your thigh muscles, slowly lower into a plié, rising on your toes to aid in range of movement. Keep your arms out in front of you for balance. Rise from the plié and bring your legs together.

Position Three

Slide your right foot forward so that it is parallel to your left foot, with about 16 inches of space between your feet. Open your arms to the sides, rounding them slightly. Using your thigh muscles, slowly lower into a plié, making sure your knees extend over your toes. Allow your arms to extend out for balance. Rise from the plié and return to your starting position. You will most likely need to rise slightly on your toes to achieve depth in the plié.

Position Four

Slide your left foot forward so that it is parallel to your right foot, with about 16 inches of space between your feet. Open your arms to the sides, rounding them slightly. Using your thigh muscles, slowly lower into a plié, making sure your knees extend over your toes. Allow your arms to extend out for balance. Rise from the plié and return to your starting position. You will most likely need to rise slightly on your toes to achieve depth in the plié.

Prone Cobra

(neck, upper and middle back)

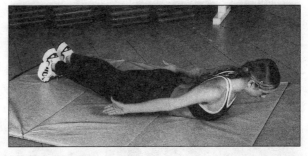

This is a beginning-level exercise to help reverse a forward head posture. It works the muscles that pull the head backward and the upper and middle back muscles that pull the shoulders back.

Lie facedown, arms to your sides, palms up. To protect your neck and lower back, it's important to keep your chin tucked in, your eyes focused on the floor, and your lower abs contracted slightly.

Begin by lifting your head and shoulders off the floor; as you do, squeeze your shoulder blades together and externally rotate your hands (turning them outward) until your thumbs point upward. Your head should be aligned with your spine—don't tilt your head down. Return to the start, internally rotating your hands so your palms face up once again.

Although lifting your shoulders off the floor will work the upper back muscles, externally rotating your hands increases the range of motion so you receive maximum benefit.

Prone Triceps Extension

(triceps)

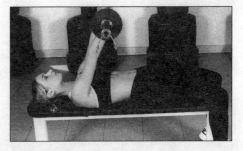

Lie faceup on a bench and hold an E-Z curl barbell with a narrow grip, palms facing away from your body. Your head should be fully supported by the bench-do not let it hang over the edge. Press the weight to arms' length to assume the start position. Keeping the upper arms stationary, bend your elbows as far as comfortable and then return to the start.

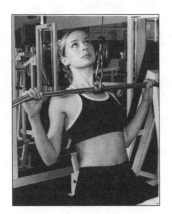

Pulldown to Chest
(upper back)

Sit on a lat pulldown machine so your torso is positioned directly underneath the cable. Sitting too far away from the machine will cause you to poke your head forward while performing the exercise, a posture that can strain your neck and upper back muscles.

Begin by pulling the bar to your collarbone, leaning slightly back until the bar touches your collarbone. Pause in this fully contracted position before slowly returning to the start.

This should be a natural movement; do not use the technique advocated by many exercise specialists in which you fully retract your shoulders and then follow through with the arms—this is especially stressful to the smaller muscles of the upper back and may eventually cause injury.

Push-Up
(arms, chest, shoulders)

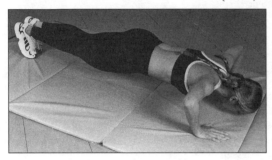

A tried and true workhorse of an exercise, the push-up is a simple but effective movement for the arms, chest and shoulders. You can use the straight-leg position, or perform the simpler version with your knees on the floor. Keeping your head in line with your spine—looking up may strain your neck—bend your arms until your chest touches the floor. Your elbows should be pointed out and slightly down. Now straighten your arms to complete the movement. Throughout the exercise keep your back as rigid as possible; do not drop or raise your hips.

If this exercise bothers your wrists or shoulders, you can experiment with special push-up handles available in many gyms and major sporting goods stores. These allow you to perform the exercise with minimal flexion of the wrists.

Rear Leg Kick
(hamstrings, buttocks, lower back)

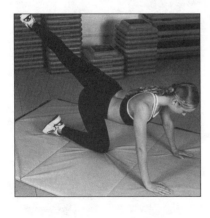

In addition to working the hamstrings and glutes, the rear leg kick is an excellent postural exercise because it strengthens the spinae erectors, the two cable-like muscles that run down the middle of the back.

Get down on all fours (knees and palms) so your upper thighs and your arms are perpendicular to the floor. Your hands should be directly under your shoulders and your head should be aligned with your spine—do not look up! This is the start position.

Perform the exercise by lifting and extending your right leg until it is parallel to the floor, although you can lift it a little higher if this does not bother your lower back. Return to the start to complete the movement. Perform all the reps for that leg before performing an equal number of reps for the other leg.

You may notice that one side of your body is usually much more stable than the other; this is perfectly normal and is often simply a result of daily lifestyle postures that create muscle imbalances. This imbalance is often quickly corrected with this exercise.

To increase the difficulty of the exercise, use ankle weights.

Reverse Crunch
(lower abdominals)

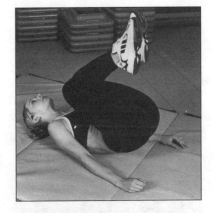

This is an excellent exercise for the lower abdominals, but only if performed correctly. It can be done lying flat on the floor or on a sturdy bench; choose the variation you find most comfortable.

Keeping your head down and hands at your sides (or holding the edges of a bench), pull your knees to your chest to assume the start position. Begin the exercise by rolling your hips so your knees move toward your head. Continue the movement to the point just before your shoulder blades would have to lift off the floor, then slowly return to the start. Throughout the exercise keep your legs tucked in. Also, if the movement feels uncomfortable on your lower back, try performing it with your hands under your buttocks.

To increase the difficulty of the exercise, perform it on an incline bench or hold a dumbbell or medicine ball between your feet.

Rowing Machine, Seated
(upper back)

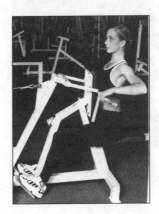

This exercise for strengthening the back muscles requires a low row machine or a low-pulley cable apparatus. Sit down and bend your knees slightly—do not lock them, as this can overstress your lower back. Keep your back slightly arched and tuck in your chin slightly.

Begin by leaning forward slightly from the hips, then pull your shoulders back while bending the arms. Your arms should be positioned a few inches away from your sides as you do this. Keep pulling, leaning backward and allowing the bar to touch the middle of your chest. At this point, finish the movement by squeezing the shoulder blades together. Return to the start.

As you perform this entire movement, keep your head in line with your torso—do not poke your head forward.

Rugby Sit-Up
(upper abdominals)

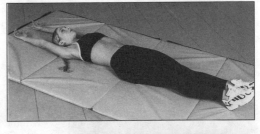

The rugby sit-up is an advanced upper abdominal exercise, and it should be performed only by those who have developed strong lower abdominal muscles. It is not as stressful as the jackknife sit-up, however, even though it likewise combines a crunch movement with a leg lift.

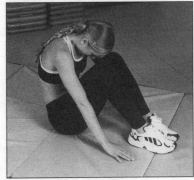

Lie on your back with your arms and legs outstretched. From this starting position pull your legs up until your feet touch the floor; as you do this, curl your trunk forward, lift your arms overhead in an arch, and touch the floor in front of you as far forward as possible. Ideally, your chest should touch your upper thighs in the finished position. From here, slowly return to the start.

If this exercise bothers your back, it may be because you lack sufficient lower abdominal (external obliques) strength to counter the pull of the hip flexor muscles. If this is the case, substitute easier upper-abdominal exercises such as the abdominal crunch.

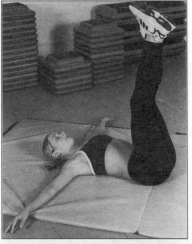

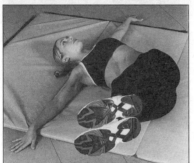

Russian Twist
(obliques)

This exercise not only strengthens the obliques but is also an effective stretch for the glutes and lower back.

Lie faceup and extend your arms out to the sides. Bring your feet together and lift them straight up until they are perpendicular to the floor. This is the start position.

Begin by allowing the legs to slowly drop to one side as far as comfortable, keeping your shoulders and head on the floor by bracing them with your arms. When you've achieved maximum stretch, return to the start and lower to the other side. Rotating to the right, then back to center, and rotating left, then back to center, equals one repetition. As for breathing, hold your breath as you lower your legs, and exhale when your legs are nearly back to center.

If this exercise performed in this manner is too difficult for you, make it easier by bending your legs and shortening your range of motion. To increase the difficulty, add ankle weights or hold a medicine ball between your ankles.

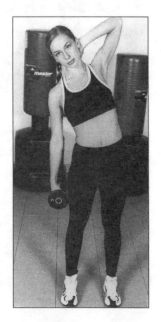

Side Bend, Dumbbell
(obliques)

Many of us have tight or weak obliques that cause postural changes in the spine that can eventually result in back pain. This is a great exercise to help resolve this problem because as it strengthens one side of the body, it stretches the other.

Hold a dumbbell in one hand and place your other hand behind your head. Without bending your knees, lower the dumbbell down your leg as far as comfortable, return to the start, then lean in the other direction. As you perform the movement do not lean forward or twist the hips. After you've completed all the reps for that side, place the dumbbell in your other hand and repeat.

When you first perform this exercise, you will probably notice you are much stronger and more flexible on one side than the other. This is normal but will be corrected quickly with this exercise. However, to avoid worsening any strength imbalance, use the same weight for both sides.

Squat, Ballet

(hips, thighs, buttocks, inner thighs)

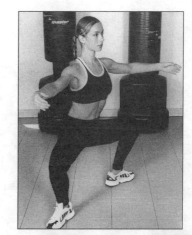

This is a variation of the squat that places extra emphasis on the inner thighs. Stand with your feet slightly wider than shoulder-width apart, feet pointed out as far as comfortable. Starting with your hands in front of you, squat down as far as comfortable, keeping your head up and torso erect, and lift your hands out to the side as shown. Return to the start.

As your strength, flexibility and stability improve, attempt to squat deeper. When you first perform this exercise you may want to stand close to a wall or other object you can use for balance.

Squat, Dumbbells

(hips, thighs, buttocks)

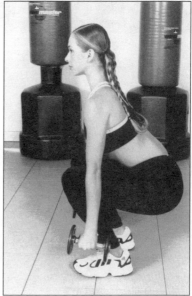

The squat is an excellent exercise for the entire lower body and, despite propaganda to the contrary, is very safe. Studies have shown that when done properly, squats actually strengthen the knee joint.

Hold a dumbbell in each hand, palms facing each other. With your feet flat on the floor, shoulder-width apart, find a point high on the wall near the ceiling and focus your eyes on it. This is your start position.

Keeping your head up and your torso as erect as possible (and only bending forward when absolutely necessary to drop further down), slowly bend your knees, allowing your knees to travel outward over your toes. Try to lower yourself so your thighs go well past parallel to the floor, but do not bottom out or bounce in the low position. Using your legs and resisting the temptation to lean forward excessively, push out of the bottom position to return to the start.

Squat, Hack, on Smith Machine

(hips, thighs, buttocks)

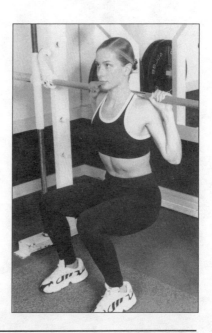

Begin with a bar resting across your shoulders in a Smith machine. Move your feet in front of the bar about a foot so that your upper back is perpendicular to the floor. With your feet flat on the floor and shoulder-width apart, find a point high on the wall near the ceiling and focus your eyes on it. Keeping your head up and your torso as erect as possible, slowly bend your legs. Try to lower yourself so your thighs go past a parallel line with the floor, but do not bottom out or bounce in the low position. Using your legs and resisting the temptation to lean excessively forward, push out of the bottom position to return to the start.

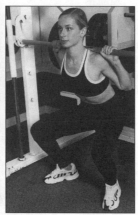

Squat, Smith Machine
(hips, thighs, buttocks)

Begin with a bar resting across your shoulders in a Smith machine. With your feet flat on the floor and shoulder-width apart, find a point high on the wall near the ceiling and focus your eyes on it. Keeping your head up and your torso as erect as possible, slowly bend your legs, allowing your knees to travel outward over your toes. Try to lower yourself so your thighs go past a parallel line with the floor, but do not bottom out or bounce in the low position. Using your legs and resisting the temptation to lean forward, push out of the bottom position to return to the start.

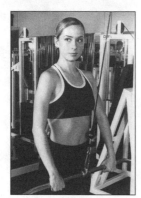

Straight-Arm Pulldown
(upper back, shoulders, triceps, abdominals)

Stand in front of a high pulley with a long bar. Stand back from the pulley so you can bend over and remain clear of the weight stack. Grasp the bar with a medium-width grip, turning your wrists down to minimize the stress on them. Bend forward at the waist, keeping your back straight and your head up. Spread your feet shoulder-width apart and keep your knees unlocked. Using a palms-down grip and keeping your arms straight and elbows locked, pull the bar down toward your knees.

This variation of the pulldown works your upper back, shoulders and triceps. It is also an excellent exercise for the abdominals; in fact, studies have shown that the upper abdominals contract harder during this type of exercise than they do during sit-ups.

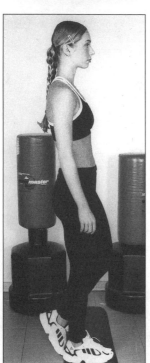

Step-Up
(thighs)

Here is a great exercise for those with bad knees. In fact, along with the Petersen step-up, this is one of the best exercises you can perform to rehabilitate your knees.

Find a sturdy box or bench, or several aerobic steps, that is high enough so that when you put one foot on it, your upper thigh is parallel to the floor. Position yourself facing the box so that the entire surface of your right foot is on the box and your left foot is on the floor, just a few inches away from the box. Point your right foot straight ahead or slightly out, whichever position you find the most stable. Pull your shoulders back and look straight ahead. This is the start position.

Perform the exercise by straightening your right leg, keeping your left foot just a few inches from the box. After straightening your right leg, slowly return to the start. Do not allow your back leg to cross behind your front leg or you may lose your balance. Continue in this manner until you have completed all the reps for that side, then switch legs.

If you feel off-balance during this exercise, step onto the box at the top of each rep.

Triceps Extension and Press

(chest, shoulders, triceps)

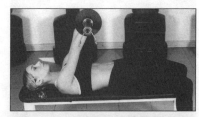

This exercise combines two sets into what is called a compound exercise. The first part isolates the triceps; the second part works the chest and shoulders. Technically it could be called a superset because you perform the two exercises in sequence, with no rest between sets.

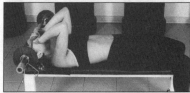

Take a close grip (hands a few inches from each other) on a light exercise bar or E-Z curl bar—the E-Z curl bar rotates your hands to minimize the stress on your wrists. Lie back on a flat bench, with the bar resting on your chest. Your head should be fully supported by the bench—do not let it hang over the edge, as this will strain your neck. Lift your upper arms so they are perpendicular to the floor, then slowly allow the forearms to travel back toward your head as far as comfortable. Pause at the stretched position, then reverse the movement to return to the start.

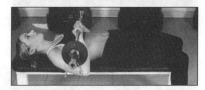

For the second exercise, begin with the bar on your chest and then press it to arms' length. Slowly return to the start, pause, then repeat. One rep of each exercise constitutes one compound rep.

Triceps Pressdown

(triceps)

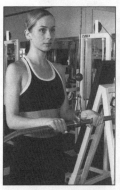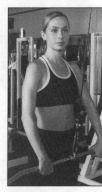

This is performed with a high-pulley apparatus such as is found on a cable crossover or lat machine, with a straight bar attachment.

Stand facing the weight stack and grasp the bar with an overhand grip. Look straight ahead, chin pulled in. Pull the bar down until your arms are parallel to the floor, elbows tucked against your sides and wrists turned down. From this start position, flex your triceps until the bar is straight, then slowly return to the start.

Upright Row, Dumbbells

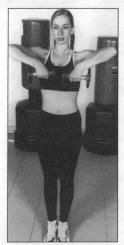

Hold two dumbbells about four inches apart, palms facing your body. Curl your wrists so that your elbows flare out to the sides. Look straight ahead and retract your chin. Begin the exercise by shrugging your shoulders and bending your arms until the dumbbells touch your collarbone. Your elbows should be coming up, not back. Now reverse the movement, returning the bar to arms' length.

If you're not able to bring the weight to your collarbone, it could be due to a lack of flexibility, but more likely, it means you're using too much weight. Also, if you have a difficult time holding on to the bar during the last few reps, use lifting straps to reinforce your grip.

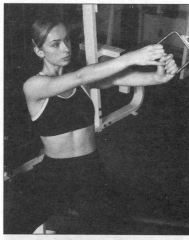

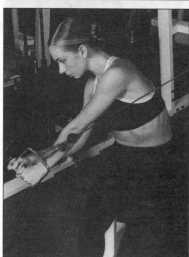

Wood Chop, Seated
(obliques)

This is an advanced exercise for the obliques that, because it is performed with a weight stack, enables you to easily increase the resistance incrementally.

Place a bench parallel with a high-pulley unit, such as that found on a cable crossover machine. Sit down with your right side nearest the weight stack. Grasp the cable handle with your left hand covering (or above) your right hand. Now straddle the bench, face forward, and hold your arms outstretched so your torso is slightly rotated to the left. The cable should be at approximately a 45-degree angle to the floor, and you should be looking at the cable handle, with your shoulders in line with your head. This is the start position.

Perform the exercise by pulling the cable handle down in a diagonal pattern, at approximately 45 degrees, with your arms straight. As you do so, follow the cable handle with your eyes and head, and rotate your shoulders and torso down to achieve a full contraction. Reverse the procedure to return to the start. After you've completed all the reps for that side, repeat for the other side, placing your right hand over your left and rotating in the opposite direction.

This may at first appear to be a complex exercise, but it really isn't—after a few sets you should have the technique mastered. However, it can be a very intense exercise, so for your first several workouts you should use especially light weights.

I hope this article is read as it was intended, to educate and inform people on certain aspects of drug use in the sport of women's bodybuilding. It was compiled from more than 30 interviews with women who have used a variety of drugs, stacks and dosages for periods ranging from three months to more than 6 years. Please don't bother trying to identify the sources: the majority of them have long since retired from the limelight, and I'd lay odds your guesses would be wrong anyway—remember, there are thousands of women who have taken steroids but have never set foot on Venice Beach nor earned a single mention in a magazine. It is to these women this article is dedicated. I hope I have shared some of their silent agony to help them know they are not alone.

The Androgen Women

*A look inside a world of women
who have used steroids*
(First printed in *Muscle Media 2000*, 1994)

by Laura Dayton

On a clear morning you can witness a spectacular sunrise from the east balcony of this sprawling California home. The first rays streak through the dewy treetops to cast their red-glow reflections across the serene surface of the pool. This is her favorite spot, although her husband prefers the breakfast nook with a steaming cup of coffee. It's the start of a good day, she thinks, letting go a little smile up towards the warm, glowing orange sun before she turns to go back inside. She's always been an early riser, which is a good thing as she sits down and scoots a stool closer to the large mirror in her well-lit bathroom. Then she begins her morning ritual of plucking her beard, whisker-by-whisker, from her face.

Not too far away, a woman sits alone in a dim room furnished with hand-me-downs and strewn with the crumpled, dog-eared copies of bodybuilding magazines. Her cheeks are hollow and her skin looks leprosied from the fading pro-tan. Her eyes are red and swollen from tears of exhaustion and depression. She looks down at her forearm, then clenches her fist so hard that the too-long fake nails bite into the skin. The muscles jump into relief, the tendons and veins stand out like worms, and a smile comes to her wan, nearly skeletal, face. Twisting the fist from side-to-side she watches the forearm flex and her bicep pop up. Suddenly her smile fades and she slams her fist down in anger and frustration, causing the cheap coffee table to buck, and the third-place trophy to tumble over with a hollow 'clack' as the plastic breaks on the hardwood floor.

In yet another city a young mother grows anxious as she watches her son throw a tantrum. The terrible twos, that's all it is, she nervously tells herself. He's big for his age. Big and strong, like his mom. The toddler picks up a toy truck and throws it against the wall. Maybe it's because he was premature; maybe he's attention deficit; maybe he'll grow out of it. She bites her lip and looks at him helplessly. Or, maybe he's this way because of the drugs she took. The worst thing is the guilt, because she'll never really know.

These three very different scenarios have one thing in common: they are all excerpts from the lives of women who have taken steroids. They are three of thousands of women who have taken drugs to earn the coveted recognition of the sport of bodybuilding. They are bodybuilders, but beyond that, they belong to a very special, very private, elite group: the androgen women. They are women who will live the rest of their lives permanently altered from the use of male hormones. They are different, yet they rarely talk about their conditions amongst each other, and almost never with an outsider. Not a doctor, a mother or a boyfriend, and least of all, the press. Until now.

Getting to the Truth

There may be a few rare exceptions, but to compete nationally and at the pro level, female bodybuilders use drugs. Steroids, estrogen blockers, thyroid drugs, growth hormone and diuretics are commonly used, sometimes alone, most often in combinations. The bulk of the side effects discussed in this article are caused by steroids, but the other drugs may be silent accomplices. Unfortunately, it is nearly impossible to ascertain which drugs or dosages are responsible for what side effect due to the fact that the black market is flooded with counterfeit and imported drugs, leaving the user guessing as to what she is really taking.

Everyone knows that drugs impart muscular size and strength. But the drugs do more than what is exploited in the gym or in a posing suit. This article is about those changes.

The drugs and dosages that women bodybuilders take are unique—they are more similar in dosage to the drugs given for gender changing from female to male than to any other therapeutic application. No legal medical procedure, with the exception of gender dysphoria treatments, administers anything close. Two medical doctors laughed when I asked their opinion on a typical bodybuilder's drug profile—they simply did not believe a human being, especially a female, was taking those dosages. Therefore, I've used for comparison and sometimes confirmation, information from gender dysphoria clinics and studies. Transsexuals going from female to male use a minimum dosage of 200 mg. of depotestosterone every two weeks, for life. I spoke with one woman bodybuilder who claimed to have used 200 mg. injections of testosterone every four days, for eight weeks. That makes what the transsexuals use look mild, but it still provided the best source of scientifically documented changes to females' secondary sexual characteristics in reaction to large doses of steroids.

Most bodybuilders would not intentionally use pure testosterone; however, it is often contained in black market drugs and injected or ingested unknowingly. Testosterone is considered to be completely androgenic, meaning that it produces only the secondary sexual characteristics. Drugs such as primobolin are considered anabolic, but no steroid is completely free of the androgenic qualities that cause male secondary sexual characteristics to develop in women. The empirical data from the transsexual studies is used for comparison and does not imply that female bodybuilders are transsexual.

Because there are no true parallels, the best source for information is the bodybuilders themselves—and therein lies the biggest stumbling block to getting at the truth. To put it bluntly, most of them lie.

"Honesty is a commodity quite lacking in bodybuilding," said one woman interviewed. "If bodybuilders get honest, they'll see that what they do isn't worth it. There's no pot of gold—I can count on one hand the pros that ever really made money. They don't face the truth about their sport, or the drugs. Especially the women, it's tough to face up to the fact that you've altered yourself for life to get a lousy trophy or to bench 165."

While the dishonesty may be a symptom of the sport, there is also evidence that it is symptomatic of drug use in general.

"A chemically altered person does not think the same as when they are not on the drugs," says Colleen Moore, program director for the drug counseling center New Connections. "When they are on a drug—whether it's amphetamines, alcohol, cocaine or steroids—they don't see the consequences of the problem. They are in a complete state of denial, and lying is very common."

Regardless of why people lie, you've got to accept that not every person interviewed was telling the whole truth, and nothing but. When more than one woman says the same thing, I would venture to say it is true. The isolated, possibly inflammatory statements, may be just that. Take them with a grain of caution.

Among the questions, each of the 32 women interviewed was asked whether she regretted the decision to use drugs. Although always preceded with a moment's hesitation, the majority said no. Three of them said the tradeoff was worth it; that bodybuilding had provided them some of the most rewarding moments of their lives. However, when asked if they could return to their pre-drug state, free of excess hair, a deepened voice and an enlarged clitoris, all but one of the women said they would go back gladly, and given a second chance, would never touch the drugs.

In the course of interviews for this article several women said, "If I only knew then, what I know now." That's exactly what you're about to read: what they know now, plus the little bit that medical science can add. It is not complete and it is not definitive. But it is the closest thing to the truth you'll ever read about women and steroids. So, if you know a woman who is just beginning to get serious about bodybuilding; if you know a woman you suspect is being tempted to use drugs; or if you know a woman who—as all the women here once believed—thinks the side effects won't happen to her, please give her this article.

The Bearded Woman

Next to the deepening of the voice, facial hair growth is the most irritating of the permanent side effects. It is a condition that occurred in all but one of the women interviewed. The exception was the woman who used drugs for only three months, but short usage is no guarantee. Two women began to get coarse facial hair during their first six-week cycle; for others it occurred several cycles into their usage, regardless of how carefully they tried to stay away from the highly androgenic drugs like testosterone and dianabol, or how small the doses they used. The extent of facial hair growth increased with dosage and duration; however, don't get the impression that steroids are producing female versions of Grizzly Adams.

Even in female-to-male transsexuals, achieving dense, full beards with regular use of testosterone is a hit-or-miss therapy. It appears that beard density is dependent on factors other than hormone levels.

The women bodybuilders experienced an increase and thickening of facial hairs, and the worst cases described it in a variety of ways:

"It's kind of like a 16- or 17-year old boy when he first starts to grow a beard. I couldn't grow sideburns and a mustache or anything."

"It's controllable with plucking, but it's definitely thick enough to consider it a beard. My eyebrows got thicker and longer, and so did the hair down the back of my neck, but it never went to my shoulders or back. My legs are real hairy too, but that could be the shaving."

"It's blonde and not really noticeable, but it's definitely not the peach fuzz it used to be. It's gross."

While on a drug cycle, the condition worsens. Off the drugs it lessens somewhat. There was no change in hair color: natural blondes had blond facial hair; brunettes had dark facial hair.

Although it is possible to stimulate hair growth on the chest and shoulders, something that is common in transsexual drug therapies, this appears to be rare in bodybuilding women, possibly due to the use of low androgenic drugs and cycling on and off, or perhaps it is determined more by genetic predisposition. A receding hairline and male pattern baldness are also possible, but appear to be rare and determined more by family history. Because male hair loss may not manifest itself until a person reaches their 40s or 50s, this condition may become a problem for these women as they age.

Most women control facial hair with plucking. Shaving is the least desirable because it leaves a visible stubble, and some women believe it worsens the situation. According to esthetician Lori Nestore, a hair removal expert featured in *Muscle and Fitness*, electrolysis is the only permanent solution, but it is not practical for dense growth.

"Electrolysis requires four or five visits per hair, and

the number of hairs worked on in any given visit is dependent on a person's pain tolerance," says Nestore. "This would be a practical solution only for those with sparse facial hair. I wouldn't recommend waxing the face because the stubble that must grow between waxes would not be acceptable to women. A combination of some electrolysis and plucking is the best way to deal with it."

Clitoral Enlargement and Sexual Appetites

Like facial hair, some degree of clitoral enlargement occurred in all the women interviewed, with the single exception the woman who used drugs for only three months. Again, it can't be assumed that short-duration drug use won't cause clitoral growth. Clitoral growth was gradual and most of the women couldn't recall with accuracy when it began, but several said they noticed a change early.

Enlargement was most commonly described as "noticeably bigger than before, but not so big that I can't wear a swimsuit, posing suit or tights." The most growth reported in this survey was described as "about the length of half my little pinky." Or, nearly an inch and one-half.

In transsexual studies, one and three-quarter inches was common after one year of testosterone therapy; the longest reported was two and two-thirds inches.

Clitoris enlargement is greatest when using drugs and diminishes when off drugs. Sensitivity is also increased, but the degree varied greatly.

"It drove me crazy," said one woman. "It was rubbing against everything and it was incredibly sensitive. It was really tough to ignore."

Along with the heightened sensitivity, some, but not all, reported an increased sexual appetite. Some of these women mentioned increased aggression and easier, more intense orgasms. Sexual behavior seemed to be dictated more by the woman's previous sexual appetites than by the drugs. No one felt the increased aggressiveness was out of control or would lead to indiscriminate sex, and no one reported sexual attraction toward other women.

Several women reported a decrease in sexual arousal when off the drugs. They were not certain if sexual drive decreased below their pre-drug level. Women with greater enlargement reported a problem with excess skin, and noticed increased difficulty achieving orgasm. One woman described it as a "foreskin." Several women expressed interest in surgery to remove the excess skin, but were at a loss as to where to go to obtain it. In phone calls to several plastic surgeons, it appears that the surgery can be performed but would carry an inherent risk of accidental castration because surgeons do not have any experience performing this type of operation.

The Baritone Voice

This was the most irritating, embarrassing and unwanted side effect. It was experienced by approximately two-thirds of the women interviewed. All the women who had knowingly taken testosterone and highly androgenic drugs had a deepening of the voice, but so did some who swore they had only used the mildest, least androgenic drugs. Those who didn't

experience a voice change attributed it to low dosage and mild drugs.

In one case, the voice was affected only two weeks into her first cycle. Other women said it was over a period of months. Several of the women changed the drugs they were using as soon as the voice deepening began, but the damage was done. As with the other side effects, the voices were deepest while on the drugs, but resumed some of their former resonance when the drugs were discontinued. One woman reported that the change to the vocal chords made speech painful and it was difficult to make herself heard in crowded rooms or to shout. Three women lamented that prior to the drug use they had enjoyed singing at octaves they could no longer achieve.

Several women had inquired about surgeries to scrape the vocal chords, but none had undergone the procedure because they had all heard the operation had less than satisfactory results. One physician I interviewed had performed the operation, and he agreed that the surgery has a low success rate and that it is nearly impossible to restore a voice to its former quality.

Emotional Roller Coasters

Women: Imagine your worst bout of PMS ever. That's par for the course if you decide you want to use bodybuilding drugs.

"As for the emotional side, I don't think I was so bad, but if you asked my husband you'd get a different story!

"There is so much that goes on with the dieting, and the training, and it just takes over your whole life. I think anyone would have thrown the bathroom scale across the room, drugs or not!"

"I was zingin', man. I mean ups and downs like you wouldn't believe. I tried to off myself. It was bad. Real bad."

"I think the toughest part was coming off the drugs. When you lose the strength and start to smooth out. It was depressing."

"When I was on the stuff I thought I was superwoman. It was really amazing. Totally amazing. It improved my self-esteem immensely. That's something that I won't regret."

"I guess I was lucky because my drugs were physician-prescribed. One of the things he gave me was Parlodel, an anti-depressant, but I never understood why he gave me that."

That answer lies in the fact that steroids are hormones, and hormones affect a person's emotions. Every woman is familiar with monthly mood swings; now imagine them magnified 10, 20, 30 and 40 times.

Back in the 80s, there was a national-level competitor who picked up a gun and blew her brains out. Rumor said it was a bad drug comedown. No one knows for certain. Several of the women interviewed felt there is too much made of steroid-induced depression, and that if someone commits suicide, they would be just as predisposed to self-destruction with or without the drugs.

All the women experienced increased aggression and short tempers, but many admitted it could have been the diet or other factors. There appears to be a definite increase in aggression, no matter how mild the drugs or dosage, or how short the duration of drug use. The aggression and anger dissipated when the drugs were discontinued.

Bodybuilders and Babies

Here is where we get into some real gray territory. Interestingly, nearly half the women interviewed had told their gynecologists about their drug use; however, they hadn't learned one iota more about their conditions than the women who never asked. The bottom line is that nobody knows exactly what happens to a woman's reproductive system.

All the women interviewed stopped menstruating when they used the drugs. All their periods returned when they stopped the drugs, some within weeks, some within months. Some women went back to a regular cycle, some did not. Some women got pregnant, some did not (but they also weren't trying). No woman knew of any permanent effects to her reproductive system.

Judy Van Maasdam, program director for the Gender Dysphoria clinic at Stanford University, said that transsexuals receiving testosterone treatments resume their periods when the drugs are stopped, even after several years of ongoing therapy. However, she said it is suspected that longer use or excessively higher doses and/or combinations of hormones could permanently suppress circulating hormones and prevent ovulation. Studies by the University of Texas indicated that it would require a testosterone concentration above 1000 ng/dl to suppress FSH (follicle stimulating hormone), a blood concentration high even by bodybuilding standards.

Women who are uncertain of their fertility should consult a gynecologist for a FSH test. This is the same test used to determine if menopause has occurred. If the test comes back negative, indicating that the woman is no longer ovulating, she should periodically repeat the test if she is in her childbearing years. Steroid use should never be used as a form of birth control. It is possible to ovulate—and get pregnant— even in the absence of a regular menstrual cycle.

It appears that women who use steroids can get pregnant. However, there is speculation—not proof or even documented evidence, but speculation—that steroid use may have effects upon children. A woman's ovaries do not produce eggs—they store them. A woman is born with all her eggs, therefore, all her eggs are present when she uses the drugs. It is known that the ovaries come equipped with powerful hormone-sensitive receptors. It is not known whether previous steroid use can affect an unborn child.

Using steroids while pregnant is another story. Studies on female rhesus monkeys showed that when given male hormones early in their pregnancies, they gave birth to female offspring that exhibited increased aggression and enlarged clitorises, and the labia majora were partially fused, seemingly to form a scrotal sack.

Of the women interviewed who had children, all of them expressed some concern that their drug use may have had an effect, as yet unseen, on their children.

Only one woman said she noticed anything uncommon or out of the ordinary in her child. That woman had a son who she said was abnormally large and aggressive in his behavior. Medical doctors had not diagnosed any problems and there is no proof that the child's size or aggression had anything to do with the mother's history of steroid use.

Liver and Endocrine Function

None of the women interviewed were aware of any internal disorders or problems. To the contrary, several women said they never had a problem with high blood pressure or cholesterol. However, scientific research indicates that steroid use has the potential for liver damage, raising cholesterol levels and cardiovascular damage.

A study on transsexuals, published in the *Archives of Sexual Behavior*, vol. 15, 1986, indicated that cholesterol and triglyceride levels rose with increased doses of testosterone, leading researchers to the conclusion that coronary heart disease risk could increase. This, however, was based on continuous use of testosterone.

Taking any kind of hormone affects a person's endocrine system. One woman reported that after going off a particularly heavy cycle, she began lactating and found herself in the gym with milk literally squirting from her breasts. Although she has never found a medical explanation, she continues to suffer from endocrine problems and has trouble with severe mood swings when using even the lowest dosages of birth control pills.

Many of the women reported abnormalities in their periods after using drugs, but were not certain if these were caused by the drugs or by a low level of body fat. Every woman who had given birth reported that following the pregnancy, her hormones evened out and she began menstruating regularly.

The Shape and Skin of the Body

All the women reported drastic increases in muscle size, density, hardness and strength. Although there was a decrease in muscle size and strength when they got off the drugs, no woman ever went back to her original proportions. Interestingly, transsexuals do not experience muscle growth in the absence of weight training. This may make a case for weight training, or for the use of the anabolic drugs over testosterone.

Of the women who no longer trained and were trying to un-muscle their bodies, the arms were reported to be the hardest muscle to lose.

"The legs are the first to go, then the delts, then the back. But the arms, I may have these till the day I die."

Many of the women reported a change in their body type, going from lean and lithe, to stocky and blocky.

"I was always thin and small," said one woman who at 5-foot-2 now weighs 155. "I knew I'd gain weight when I started the drugs—that's what I wanted: more muscle. But somehow, because women are used to gaining and losing pounds all their lives, I just assumed in the back of my mind that I'd be able to lose the extra weight if I wanted. That's not what happened; instead, when I got off, I just kept getting bigger and bigger. I used to wear a size 6; now the best I could hope for is to squeeze into a size 10. And it's not all fat either, most of it's muscle. I just turned into a big person."

"It changes your metabolism," said another. "I used to be like a rabbit, I could eat anything. Now, everything I touch turns to fat. I hate it."

The good news is that after getting pregnant, metabolisms returned to their previous fat-eating modes and the women reported gaining back their more feminine shapes—in body and face.

Several women reported a squaring of the jawline and "hardness" in the facial contours while using drugs. In most of these cases, the facial contours went back to "nearly" normal when the drug use was discontinued. According to Van Maasdam of Stanford's Gender Dysphoria clinic, the hormones are not responsible for a change in contours of the face, but definitely to the skin.

"From what I've seen over the years, use of male hormones can age the skin," said Van Maasdam. "It becomes coarser and rougher, and that gives the face a more masculine look, but the hormones don't actually change the bone contours."

Growth hormone is the drug responsible for the severe masculinizing of the jaw and brow apparent on some women. This is because growth hormone can cause bone to resume growth. It also speeds up metabolism, and is theorized to be the drug responsible for the harder look of the top ten Ms. Olympia contestants this year.

"180 pounds and ripped—that's a big woman. You can't tell me they aren't doing some pretty serious stuff," commented one of the women interviewed about the latest Ms. Olympia.

No one in this interview admitted using growth hormone. Several related that they believed growth hormone is not responsible for the side effects of facial hair, clitoris enlargement and deepened voice, but that is a moot point since steroids must be used for growth hormone to be effective.

Acne is a problem. On the drugs, women reported gross, pustule acne on their faces, shoulders, back, chest and arms. Oily skin types were more susceptible, as was anyone with a predisposition for acne.

"It was like I was 13 all over again, but worse," said one of several women who still bear the acne scars. "Like the other side effects, you think that it's not going to happen to you. But it does, and as with all the side effects, it permanently alters you for life."

In addition to acne, enlarged pores are a common complaint. When the drugs were stopped, most of the acne cleared up, but women still complained of large pores. Skin peels can be effective to correct this condition.

Surprisingly, it does not appear that loss of breast size is a byproduct of the drugs. Breast size decreased on all the women who had large breasts to begin with, but it correlated with a general loss in body fat. Transsexuals who undergo testosterone treatment do not lose breast size, according to the University of Texas study.

The Final Chapter

"People have asked why I don't do the Olympia, and it's because I don't want to do what those women are doing. You've got to draw the line."

"I used to be one of the biggest women. Now I'm dwarfed on stage. The drug testing is a joke."

"I will not do what it takes to win the Olympia. Nope. No way."

These and other comments repeated themselves throughout these interviews. The "what" the women are doing at the Ms. Olympia contest was somewhat nebulous. Growth hormone certainly, and excessively high doses of steroids. Whatever they are doing, it's agreed by many that the Ms. Olympia has finally crossed the line into the realm of an all-out freak show. As George Snyder, founder of the first Ms. Olympia, says, "they have become he-shes. They are more men than women." Indeed, while they are on the drugs that may be true. And sadly, once off the drugs, they are never the same.

But the final chapter has not been written—a pendulum needs to complete its widest arc before it can come to rest somewhere in the middle. Women's bodybuilding continues to exist at a local level, where more women are choosing to just say no. These women prefer the more muscular look and athletic bent of a bodybuilding contest over a fitness contest. They love to train, and train hard. At the least, by establishing a more open forum regarding drugs and what they do to women, women will be able to make their choices more informed and aware of the risks.

Hopefully, this is the start of a new and more informed era of women's bodybuilding, and not the end.

*L*aura Dayton, of Napa, California, has been an integral force in the development of women's fitness programs since the early 1970s. As editor of *Fit* and *Strength Training for Beauty* magazines she shaped the world of women and weights. In 1994 her book *Freestyle Training* sent shock waves through the industry with its unique methods for weight training for weight loss, not size. Her *Freestyle Certificate Program* and now her *Lower Body Solution Certificate Program* have reached more than 40,000 personal trainers throughout the U.S.

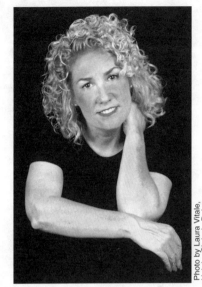

Photo by Laura Vitale.
Hair by Chrissie DeLaca

Laura has a B.A. in journalism and M.S. in mass communications. She has worked more than 25 years as a fitness journalist writing for both men's and women's fitness-related publications. She is the author of more than 1,223 articles on fitness, sports and health published in a variety of fitness-related periodicals. She is presently the owner of Dayton Publications and Writers Group in Napa, California.

She is a lifetime fitness enthusiast. She is also a lecturer on women's fitness and midlife issues. She hails from a family of bodybuilders, runners and martial artists. This book is dedicated to her husband, Chuck Drake, and her two stepkids Ashley and Jonathan, who patiently put up with yet another book project.

Other Books
and Instructional Courses
from Dayton Publications

Dayton Publications and Writers Group
1541 Third Street
Napa, California 94559
Telephone: (707) 257-2348
Fax (707) 257-2349
E-Mail: Daytonpubs@aol.com